Moral Problems
in Nursing

PHILOSOPHY AND SOCIETY
General Editor: Marshall Cohen

Also in this series:

Moral Problems
in Nursing
A Philosophical
Investigation

JAMES L. MUYSKENS

ROWMAN AND LITTLEFIELD
Totowa, New Jersey

First published in the United States 1982 by Rowman and Littlefield,
81 Adams Drive, Totowa, New Jersey 07512.

Library of Congress Cataloging in Publication Data

Muyskens, James L., 1942-
 Moral problems in nursing.

 (Philosophy and society)
 Bibliography: p.
 Includes index.
 1. Nursing ethics. I. Title. II. Series.
RT85.M83   174'.2   82-419
ISBN 0-8476-7068-6   AACR2
ISBN 0-8476-7071-6 (pbk.)

Printed in the United States of America

To Alda

Contents

Preface

For the nursing profession, the last decade has been both the best of times and the worst of times. Registered nurses have far greater responsibility than ever before. They are running cardiac monitors and respirators, operating specialized dialysis centers, oncology divisions and burn units, while remaining the mainstay of hospital care. The demand for skilled nursing care is greater than anyone would have predicted a decade ago. Yet there is great dissatisfaction in the ranks due to (among other things) a sense of a lack of autonomy on the wards, a perception of physician disrespect, low salaries, grueling and disruptive work schedules, and limited opportunity for advancement. Many of the best nurses are fleeing the profession—often leaving overcrowded floors to the inexperienced and inadequately trained.

More than ever, those entering the profession and those remaining in it feel the need to look critically at what they are doing. They are asking what they *ought* to do in the face of new and awesome responsibilities, changing conceptions of the nurse's role, job "burn out," overcrowded and understaffed health care facilities, and so on. This need has been addressed by nurses, nurse educators, philosophers, lawyers, physicians, and many others; in recent years, a large body of literature concerned with ethical issues in nursing and general health care has been produced. This book, written by a philosopher, is especially designed to help the nurse and nursing student to clarify the ethical issues confronting those in the profession today and to offer a consistent position on the many moral issues to be discussed.

As one looks at the current literature, including anthologies in bioethics and case studies in nursing, one can readily get the false impression that the way to resolve the question of what one ought to do is to decide on a course of action and then pick and choose (from among three or four) the ethical theory or approach that best supports

ix

the decision. This is not the way moral questions are to be resolved. *Moral Problems in Nursing* is intended not only as a corrective to this mistaken and dangerous view but also as an example of how one must take a moral stance that is backed by a theory and then consistently address each problem from that perspective. In short, this is a discussion of ethics for nurses and nursing students in which a point of view is taken and defended.

My hope is that the book will help the reader gain greater clarity concerning how "ought" questions are to be handled and will challenge him or her to examine critically the position advanced. The basic aim is to encourage critical reasoning about the ethical issues nurses face. I believe that the best way to begin thinking critically and developing one's own position is by working through the carefully developed position of another. This beginning point I have tried to provide. Given these goals, I will be far happier, in the end, if the reader develops his or her own well-reasoned position in opposition to mine than that mine simply is adopted uncritically. Of course, the ideal would be that readers' critical reflection would lead them to the viewpoint advanced here. The agreement of independent thinkers is one of the most effective ways of validating a point of view.

This discussion of ethics is written for both the nursing student, for whom many of the issues may be new, and the nurse for whom none are. It does not presuppose any philosophical background. The book can be read on one's own or in a course with an instructor's guidance. It can serve as the basic textbook in a course or, perhaps more effectively, as a supplement to any of the standard anthologies. Instructors of courses that include students from a variety of disciplines with varying career aspirations may want to assign it as supplementary reading for the nursing students in the class so that they can see how the topics discussed are related to the special concerns and problems of nursing.

Acknowledgments

I wish especially to thank Elsie Bandman, Ed.D., of the Bellevue School of Nursing, for her encouragement and guidance early on; Andrea Cohen, R.N., for providing me with a case study used in Chapter 4 as well as helpful comments on various issues discussed in the book; Rick Moody, Ph.D., of the Brookdale Center on Aging, for his comments on several chapters as well as use of a case study in Chapter 8; Philip Pecorino, Ph.D, of Queensboro Community College, for his helpful criticisms of an earlier version of the manuscript and for supplying me with a case study used in Chapter 5; and Phyllis Turk, R.N., C.N.M., for providing me with valuable references and discussing many of the ideas developed in the book. I owe special gratitude to the staff at Littlefield, Adams and Company, including Jim Feather, who proposed that I write this book, and Janet Johnston, who provided invaluable assistance at the final stages.

Permission from publishers to use material contained in this volume is gratefully acknowledged.

1. Extracts from Stewart Alsop, "The Right to Die with Dignity." By permission of Marie Rodell—Frances Collin Literary Agency. Copyright © 1974 by Stewart Alsop. Reprinted from *Good Housekeeping* Magazine.

2. ANA *Code for Nurses*. Published by the American Nurses' Association. Reprinted with the permission of ANA.

3. Extracts from Mary Ann Carroll and Richard A. Humphrey, *Moral Problems in Nursing: Case Studies*. Copyright © 1979 by the University Press of America, Inc., P.O. Box 19101, Washington, D.C. 20036. Reprinted by permission, all rights reserved.

4. Extracts from Terry Daniels, "The Nurse's Tale." Copyright © 1979 by News Group Publications, Inc. Reprinted with the permission of *New York* Magazine.

5. Extracts from Anne J. Davis and Mila A. Aroskar, *Ethical Dilemmas and Nursing Practice.* Copyright © 1978 by Appleton-Century-Crofts. Printed with permission.

6. Case Studies in Bioethics from the *Hastings Center Report.* Copyright © Institute of Society, Ethics and the Life Sciences, 360 Broadway, Hastings-on-Hudson, N.Y. 10706. Reprinted with permission of the Hastings Center.

7. Extracts from Barbara Tate, *The Nurse's Dilemma.* Copyright © 1977 by the International Council of Nurses, Geneva, Switzerland. Reprinted by permission of ICN.

8. Extracts from Robert M. Veatch, *Case Studies in Medical Ethics.* By permission of Harvard University Press. Copyright © 1977 by Robert M. Veatch.

9. Chapter 7 is a somewhat modified version of "Nurses' Collective Responsibility and the Strike Weapon," which appeared in *The Journal of Medicine and Philosophy,* vol. 7, no. 1. Copyright © 1982 by D. Reidel Publishing Co. I thank the *Journal* for their permission.

10. Chapter 6 is a somewhat modified version of "Collective Responsibility and the Nursing Profession" (copyright © 1978 by James L. Muyskens), which appeared initially in Thomas A. Mappes and Jane S. Zembaty, *Biomedical Ethics* (New York: McGraw-Hill Book Company, 1981).

Introduction

You have come to know your 59-year-old cancer patient quite well. Her physician has informed her that her prognosis is very poor and has urged chemotherapy as a last resort. You approach the patient with the drug and notice that she has been crying. She says she is apprehensive about the drug; she gave consent because her son wanted her to. She then tells you how she had controlled her leukemia for twelve years with natural foods and a deep belief that she should rely on God and He would provide. She asks you about alternative methods of cancer treatment such as nutrition, herbs, touch therapy, and laetrile. You discuss these with her and inform her that these methods are not sanctioned by the medical profession. Your patient is very grateful to you for taking the time to talk with her and let her share with you her apprehension. She asks you to return in the evening to talk to her son and daughter-in-law. What ought you to do?

Your patient is under her physician's care and has consented to a course of treatment. Her family is eager for her to undergo the prescribed therapy. Yet your patient or client has reservations. You consult the "Patients' Bill of Rights," which says that a patient has a right to genuine informed consent. You doubt that her decision is truly informed and truly free (uncoerced). You consider the various claims you have heard that nurses should be patient advocates. You reflect on your own professional codes of ethics (see Chapter I for the full texts and discussion of both the International Code of Nursing Ethics and the American Nurses Association Code for Nurses). As you interpret these codes, you see them as favoring the model of nursing which makes the nurse's primary obligation one to her or his patient rather than to a physician or an employer. Yet you realize that it is important that the nurse and physician really work together as a team. You wonder if an evening talk with your patient and her son and daughter-in-law is compatible with being a team player. This is especially worrisome because, in this particular case, you may also have some doubts about the wisdom of chemotherapy.

In March 1976, a nurse in Twin Falls, Idaho, Ms. Jolene Tuma, found herself in the situation described. She agreed to return and talk with her patient's son and daughter-in-law. Her action angered the patient's son, who complained to the doctor. The doctor brought charges against her for acting in an "unprofessional" way in that (it was claimed) she disrupted the physician-patient relationship. The board of nursing in her state found her guilty and suspended her license for six months. The decision was appealed to the Idaho Supreme Court, which reversed the earlier decision.

(For discussion of the Jolene Tuma case, see the following: *Nursing Outlook,* September 1977, contains a letter from Ms. Tuma concerning her case and an editorial on it. Beginning in the December 1977 issue and on through March 1978, the issues of *Nursing Outlook* contain numerous letters to the editor concerning the case. The June 1979 issue (in the "News and Reports" section) reports on the Idaho Supreme Court action. A final letter on the case appears in the July 1979 issue.)

No nurse would want to go through the ordeal endured by Ms. Tuma, even if ultimately vindicated by the court. Given the complexities of nursing, the rapid evolution in our concept of a nurse, the vagueness of nurse practice acts, and the unpredictability of the law, security against law suits probably is not possible. Nor is it very rewarding to live with the avoidance of law suits or controversy as one's basic concern and guiding principle. What is rewarding is the life that results from action motivated by the desire to do the best one can in one's appointed task.

The best nurse is not necessarily the one whose actions are never questioned by a physician or challenged in a court of law. A far more basic and important quality of the good nurse—in addition to having technical knowledge and skill—is having a clear understanding of the proper role of the nurse and the relationship a nurse ought to have with her or his patients. To achieve excellence in nursing, a truly worthy objective, one must come to terms with these as well as other *moral* issues. Surely a nurse would like to avoid confrontations with physicians and with the law, but a fundamental concern would be to do what is morally right.

This book is a systematic investigation of the moral questions that inevitably arise in nursing. Its aim is to help nurses and those preparing to be nurses to deal effectively with moral dilemmas such as that faced by Ms. Tuma. At the time of a crucial decision it is too late to reflect on the moral implications of the various possible alternative courses of action. One must act, often quickly and decisively. Prior reflection, however, can help one to respond in a way that one can be proud of later. It can help us to develop the moral sensitivity that will dispose us to act in the morally proper way.

In the case presented, one's decision is likely to be a better one if, prior to the time of choice, there has been systematic, careful reflection on issues such as the following:

i. The role of the nurse. To whom does the nurse owe primary allegiance, the patient or the physician?

ii. The nurse-physician relationship. Should the nurse-patient relationship always (ever, sometimes) be ancillary to the doctor-patient relationship? Why?

iii. The requirement of informed consent. What conditions must be satisfied for a patient's (client's) consent to be informed and free? What should the nurse's role be in either obtaining informed consent or verifying that it has been obtained?

Issues such as these, as well as the following, will be addressed in this book:

iv. When, if ever, may the nurse coerce the client or decide for him or her?

v. Must the nurse always tell the truth? What if telling the truth would, in the nurse's judgment, cause the client harm?

vi. Is it morally permissible for a nurse to join with her or his colleagues in a strike for better wages and working conditions?

vii. What are a nurse's moral obligations to the dying patient or the defective newborn?

Sometimes questions such as these are said to be unanswerable. There is some truth in this. If we are looking for answers the way we look for answers to problems in mathematics, there are no answers. Yet we can all recognize that some answers given to these fundamental questions about how nurses ought to behave are better than others. As we reflect on these questions we find that they compel us to work toward greater understanding rather than toward a neat formula for their resolution. The aim of this book is to provide some guidance for your life-long odyssey toward greater understanding.

1

Philosophical and Ethical Foundations

The Urgency of Moral Discussion in Nursing

The concern about moral questions in nursing is by no means a recent phenomenon. For as long as there have been practicing nurses there has been reflection on the ethical assumptions and implications of the care being offered. For a variety of reasons, however, moral reflection has taken on a greater urgency in recent years. Perhaps the primary reason for the prevailing sense of urgency is that we feel far less sure than we did in the past about what ought to be done.

What we ought to do is often determined to a large extent by our roles in society, whether they be those of parent, teacher, banker, nurse, police officer, and so on, or any combination thereof. When, as is presently the case in nursing, the role is rapidly changing and there is no clear consensus concerning the scope of its responsibilities and its limitations, it is very difficult to know what one's duties are. A nurse cannot, for example, simply do what is expected—frequently these days there are no clear expectations. Nor can a nurse *qua* nurse avoid having to take a stand, for she or he faces forced options. Deciding not to report a physician's error or not to sound the alert to resuscitate an elderly patient or not to agree to a request to discuss unorthodox alternative cancer therapies with a patient are as much decisions as deciding to do these things. To make decisions of this nature wisely, it is necessary to have engaged in moral reflection before being confronted by the forced option.

In addition to the uncertainty created by the changing nature of the role of the nurse, a topic to be discussed in Chapter 2, the wider range of possibilities for patient care made available by new technology makes it difficult to discern what we ought to do. A few years ago we could not keep people alive on respirators or produce "test tube babies." Deformed and mentally disabled children, who earlier would have died at birth, can now be kept alive. These new capabilities force us to re-examine issues we could take for granted in the past: What is meant by life and death? What is it to be human? In new situations brought about by technological development old ways of thinking about moral issues are no longer adequate.

Nurses are constantly agonizing over cases of clients who suffer from painful illnesses which earlier would have resulted in swift, sure deaths. Now it is possible to keep these people alive with the aid of technology, such as respirators. In many cases, however, the client continues to live but with greatly diminished mental and physical capacity. What ought the nurse to do in such situations to assist the patient? Would it ever be morally right, for example, to "pull the plug"? Sensationalistic reports of nurses who have acted on their convictions that they ought to assist their clients in this way occasionally appear in the newspapers. Sober, systematic reflection on these cases reveals how puzzling they really are.

Suppose you believe in the sanctity of human life. How is your basic principle to be applied in situations when you do not know whether your client is, in fact, dead or alive? Has your client passed beyond the point of being human? Suppose you do not feel it is necessary to maintain a life by "extraordinary means." Is the respirator an extraordinary means, or in cases such as the one you face is it an ordinary means? Suppose you do not believe in *actively* taking a person's life. Would turning off the respirator be a case of active or merely passive killing?

Especially because of many more options available as a result of the new technology, easy answers are just not satisfactory. Careful investigation of the basic principles one ought to follow is more urgent than ever. Clarification of key concepts, such as "sanctity of life," "extraordinary means," "active versus passive killing," is a prerequisite to their use in solving moral dilemmas. Knowledge of the actual situations in which the nurse finds herself or himself as well as an understanding of the various options available are necessary in order to apply the basic principles to everchanging circumstances and possibilities.

Professional codes of ethics are designed to provide the nurse with some moral guidance. They are a good place to begin our search for basic principles and for clarification of key moral concepts.

The Professional Codes

Two professional codes of ethics of primary significance for nurses practicing in the United States are the *International Code of Nursing Ethics* and the American Nurses Association *Code for Nurses*. These codes set the boundaries and outline the ideals for proper nursing practice. They embody the collective wisdom of the members of the associations which engendered them. Hence they provide us with a very good starting point for an investigation of some of the major moral problems in nursing.

The *International Code of Nursing Ethics* (which follows) was adopted by the International Council of Nurses in 1953.*

Professional nurses minister to the sick, assume responsibility for creating a physical, social and spiritual environment which will be conducive to recovery, and stress the prevention of illness and promotion of health by teaching and example. They render health-service to the individual, the family, and the community and coordinate their services with members of other health professions.

Service to mankind is the primary function of nurses and the reason for the existence of the nursing profession. Need for nursing service is universal. Professional nursing service is therefore unrestricted by considerations of nationality, race, creed, color, politics, or social status.

Inherent in the code is the fundamental concept that the nurse believes in the essential freedoms of mankind and in the preservation of human life.

The profession recognises that an international code cannot cover in detail all the activities and relationships of nurses, some of which are conditioned by personal philosophies and beliefs.

1. The fundamental responsibility of the nurse is threefold: to conserve life, to alleviate suffering, and to promote health.

2. The nurse must maintain at all times the highest standards of nursing care and of professional conduct.

3. The nurse must not only be well prepared to practise but must maintain her knowledge and skill at a consistently high level.

4. The religious beliefs of a patient must be respected.

5. Nurses hold in confidence all personal information entrusted to them.

6. A nurse recognises not only the responsibilities but the limitations of her or his professional functions; recommends or gives medical treatment without medical orders only in emergencies, and reports such action to a physician at the earliest possible moment.

7. The nurse is under an obligation to carry out the physician's orders intelligently and loyally and to refuse to participate in unethical procedures.

8. The nurse sustains confidence in the physician and other members of the health team; incompetence or unethical conduct of associates should be exposed but only to the proper authority.

*The *International Code of Nursing Ethics* has now been replaced by the *Code for Nurses*, which is now the official document for the International Council of Nurses.

9. A nurse is entitled to just remuneration and accepts only such compensation as the contract, actual or implied, provides.

10. Nurses do not permit their names to be used in connection with the advertisement of products or with any other form of self-advertisement.

11. The nurse cooperates with and maintains harmonious relationships with members of other professions and with her or his nursing colleagues.

12. The nurse in private life adheres to standards of personal ethics which reflect credit upon her profession.

13. In personal conduct nurses should not knowingly disregard the accepted patterns of behavior of the community in which they live and work.

14. A nurse should participate and share responsibility with other citizens and other health professions in promoting efforts to meet the health needs of the public—local, state, national and international.

The following, latest version of the American Nurses Association *Code for Nurses* was adopted by that body in 1976.

1. The nurse provides services with respect for human dignity and the uniqueness of the client, unrestricted by considerations of social or economic status, personal attributes, or the nature of health problems.

2. The nurse safeguards the client's right to privacy by judiciously protecting information of a confidential nature.

3. The nurse acts to safeguard the client and the public when health care and safety are affected by the incompetent, unethical, or illegal practice of any person.

4. The nurse assumes responsibility and accountability for individual nursing judgments and actions.

5. The nurse maintains competence in nursing.

6. The nurse exercises informed judgment and uses individual competence and qualifications as criteria in seeking consultation, accepting responsibilities, and delegating nursing activities to others.

7. The nurse participates in activities that contribute to the ongoing development of the profession's body of knowledge.

8. The nurse participates in the profession's efforts to implement and improve standards of nursing.

9. The nurse participates in the profession's efforts to establish and maintain conditions of employment conducive to high quality nursing care.

10. The nurse participates in the profession's efforts to protect the public from misinformation and misrepresentation and to maintain the integrity of nursing.

11. The nurse collaborates with members of the health professions and other citizens in promoting community and national efforts to meet the health needs of the public.

Similarities as well as some differences become apparent when these two codes are compared. A few of these will be noted here; others will be discussed in later chapters. Neither code is very lengthy. This has to do with their primary purpose, which is to provide a concise statement of the principles that should guide a nurse's actions. A long and cumbersome statement is a poor action guide. A price of brevity is a certain degree of vagueness and generality, another characteristic that is descriptive of both codes. We can much more readily obtain agreement on vague and general principles than on specific ones. The high degree of vagueness and generality of these codes probably has something to do with the fact that they are the products of the deliberation and votes of numerous committees and the general membership of the associations. It may be impossible to obtain agreement on more specific, controversial principles. The difficulty that arises from settling for principles as broad and general as these is in the area of applicability to specific situations. Consider, for example, the second principle of the ANA *Code for Nurses,* the principle of confidentiality. What guidance does it give in the following situation?

A nurse was caring for a patient who was being treated for a back injury. The treatment was conservative and surgery had not been suggested. The treatment was carried out for many days and included physical therapy. The progress was slow. The pain returned regularly and the increase in activity was very slow.

This once-energetic and hard-working man became very depressed by what he saw as his progress or lack of it. He did not have the patience to continue the treatment. He felt that at best his physical activity would be limited, compared to that to which he was accustomed.

During a conversation with the nurse, he mentioned he was contemplating suicide, the only solution he could see to his problem. As soon as he had voiced this plan, he immediately asked the nurse to be absolutely silent and not tell anyone of this thoughts [Tate, 1977, p. 20].

Because of its vagueness, the code could be appealed to in a defense of reporting the patient's conversation as well as in one for not reporting it. But giving support for both of the opposing courses of action amounts to no guidance at all. We are no closer to knowing which course of action is the one that "judiciously protects" the confidential information.

Suppose that the issue is decided by saying that the nurse must tell the physician because he or she is privy to any information obtained by the nurse. (I have found that this is a favored solution when the case is presented for class discussion.) It is important to see that this principle concerning the relationship between the nurse and the physician takes us beyond the code. So, if we appeal to it, it is no longer the code that is providing us guidance. If in turn we ask why we should accept this (questionable) principle, we must reflect on the nature of the nurse-physician relationship (as we shall do in Chapter 3). This example shows that the codes offer a good point of departure, but that they must be supplemented by the kind of systematic reflection in which philosophers engage.

It would be unreasonable to expect a code to do justice to every situation a nurse will face. In some situations it will be logically impossible to meet all the requirements of a code; the code cannot provide a way to solve these problems. Consider the following case: your patient is a twelve-year-old cancer victim who is suffering intense pain. She has had chemotherapy and surgery. The best medical prognosis is that she can be expected to live no more than three to six weeks. Suppose you work in a facility that has developed a team concept of patient care. You meet with all the other health professionals on the case and the patient's parents to discuss what should be done. Some members of the team recommend doing one more surgical procedure on the outside chance it would help. Others want to stop treatment and increase the narcotic dosage—although that would run the serious risk of respiratory depression and could even hasten death. Another group wants to continue modest treatment and not increase the narcotic dosage. You are unclear as to which of these suggested courses of action is best. You want to do what is morally correct.

You happen to have the *International Code of Nursing Ethics* available, so you look at it. You see that "the fundamental responsibility of the nurse is threefold: to conserve life, to alleviate suffering, and to promote health." What you want to do in this situation is to follow your professional code. You quickly discover that is impossible in this situation. If you alleviate suffering, you run a great risk of failing to conserve life. If you aim to conserve life, you cannot alleviate the suffering with high narcotic doses. If you opt for the long-shot of additional surgery to try to promote health, you fail to alleviate suffering and may actually hasten death. You discover that each of the three proposals for action takes one of these threefold responsibilities and gives it priority over the others. You realize that the question of ordering these principles is the crucial one; but the code is unable to help you with it.

One of the aims of philosophical ethics is to help us think through the question of the ordering of our moral principles. Ethical theories which philosophers devise are attempts to demonstrate that one or a few moral principles are the fundamental ones and all others are derivative from them. The reasoning involved in theory building is required to deal effectively with these conflict-of-duty situations.

Moral reasoning is also required to decide whether a code is worthy of one's adherence and which code to follow if several respected codes offer conflicting guidance. Our investigation will demonstrate that the ANA *Code for Nurses* is an excellent professional code. But to be in a position to say that, one has to develop a more-basic moral framework and criterion for moral judgment. Such a framework is also required in making decisions to follow a principle of one code rather than a conflicting or diverging one of another code.

Suppose that the nurse writing the following were trying to decide which code to follow.

I am supposed to be responsible for the control and safety of techniques used in the operating theatre. I have spent many hours teaching the technicians and the aides the routines necessary for maintaining aseptic conditions during surgery. They have learned to prepare materials and to maintain an adequate supply for all needs. They have learned to handle supplies with good technique.

I find it is extremely difficult to have these appropriate routines carried out constantly by employees with little theoretical background or understanding. The surgeons are frequently breaking techniques and respond in a belligerent manner when breaks in technique are brought to their attention. I find a reminder of techniques often brings a determined response to ignore the reminder and proceed with surgery. For a male surgeon to be questioned by a female nurse is a serious breach of respect to them.

One day a surgeon wore the same gown for two successive operations, even though there were other gowns available. I quietly called this to his attention, but I had no authority which really allowed me to control his behavior for the good of the patient. In this situation even the hospital administrator was of no help to me [Tate, 1977, pp. 47–48].

The third principle of the ANA code says: "The nurse acts to safeguard the client and the public when health care and safety are affected by the incompetent, unethical, or illegal practice of any person." The nurse's primary duty is to the client to whom she or he has a protective responsibility. Whatever is required by way of reporting the surgeon's dangerous violation of procedure must be done in the name of client welfare.

The emphasis of the complimentary principle (#8) in the *International Code of Nursing Ethics* is quite different. "The nurse sustains confidence in the physician and other members of the health team: incompetence or unethical conduct of associates should be exposed but only to the proper authority." Here the nurse's primary duty appears to be to the physician and other members of the health team. It concedes that violations should be reported. Any reporting of them, it emphasizes, must be done strictly according to protocol. Which of these principles should the nurse caught in this unfortunate situation follow? Why? To develop persuasive answers to these questions, we must pursue the investigation of fundamental moral principles that we have begun. (This case will be discussed in Chapter 6.)

In the course of her or his daily activities, a nurse comes upon ethical problems that are not covered by the codes at all. For example, neither of the codes examined says anything about whether a nurse should assist in the performance of nontherapeutic abortions, whether a nurse must always tell the truth, or whether a nurse should support a national health insurance program or participate in a strike for higher wages.

In summary, the professional codes provide an excellent starting-point from which to launch a systematic investigation of the moral problems of nursing. But because of their brevity, vagueness, generality, and incompleteness, they are not an appropriate end-point.

The Hebrew-Christian Moral Tradition

The professional codes of ethics examined have arisen out of a broader moral context, the moral tradition of our Hebrew-Christian heritage. Just as we began by *provisionally* accepting the professional codes as sound moral judgment, we shall do the same with the fundamental principle of the Hebrew-Christian moral tradition: the command to love our neighbor as ourselves. This principle is expressed in the following well-known passage in the Gospel according to Luke (10: 25–37):

And behold, a lawyer stood up to put [Jesus] to the test, saying, "Teacher, what shall I do to inherit eternal life?" He said to him, "What is written in the law? How do you read?" And he answered, "You shall love the Lord your God with all your heart, and with all your soul, and with all your strength, and with all your mind; and your neighbor as yourself." And he said to him, "You have answered right; do this, and you will live."

But he, desiring to justify himself, said to Jesus, "And who is my neighbor?" Jesus replied, "A man was going down from Jerusalem to Jericho, and he fell among robbers, who stripped him and beat him, and departed, leaving him half dead. Now by chance a priest was going down that road; and when he saw him he passed by on the other side. So likewise a Levite, when he came to the place and saw him, passed by on the other side. But a Samaritan, as he journeyed, came to where he was; and when he saw him, he had compassion, and went to him and bound up his wounds, pouring on oil and wine; then he set him on his own beast and brought him to an inn, and took care of him. And the next day he took out two denarii and gave them to the innkeeper, saying, 'Take care of him; and whatever more you spend, I will repay you when I come back.' Which of these three, do you think, proved neighbor to the man who fell among the robbers?" He said, "The one who showed mercy on him." And Jesus said to him, "Go and do likewise."

The principle expressed has two independent parts—a theological duty (to love God) and an ethical duty (to love our neighbor as ourselves). The ethical duty is a duty of respect for other persons as persons. The scope of this ethical command is broad, including all fellow human beings. The love commanded is not mere sentiment but a disposition to act in ways that express this respect. We respect others as persons when we respond to them as rational creatures as we are. Paraphrasing one of the greatest ethical thinkers of all time, Immanuel Kant (1724–1804), one must always act in ways that respect each human being (including oneself) as a creature with thoughts, plans, goals, aspirations, and hopes of one's own, that is, as a rational creature. Stating the principle in its negative form: it is impermissible to fail to treat all human beings as rational creatures. (Donagan, 1977, pp. 59–66).

Because our moral tradition has been transmitted through the ages in association with religious ones, it is common to see them as inseparable. Nevertheless, it is important to see that they are detachable. Morality can stand by itself. It is possible to accept as my obligation toward others that they be treated as rational creatures, as ends-in-themselves and not merely as means to my own ends without consideration of the question of my obligations toward God, if there be a God. Immanuel Kant's ethical theory is an attempt to demonstrate this. He argues that ethics is autonomous—meaning, in part, that it does not depend on something else, such as theological principles, for its validity. We cannot go into this deep philosophical issue here or take the time to examine Kant's arguments for his view. It is sufficient for our purposes to determine whether we find the moral principle of respect for persons to have initial plausibility as an action guide. Our answer to this question is independent of our acceptance or rejection of traditional Jewish or Christian *religious* views. One does not have to believe in the God of Abraham, Isaac, and Jacob, for example, to adopt as one's action guide the command to treat all persons as rational creatures.

The issue of the independence of theological or religious views and moral principles has a bearing on the effectiveness of moral discourse. One of the most-common reasons for engaging in a discussion of the morality of a particular action is that a conflict of interests has arisen among the affected parties. Moral principles are brought in to try to settle the conflict without resorting to such things as force, one's position of authority over the another, or personal privilege.

Suppose a patient has been acting in ways that are adversely affecting the welfare of the other patients on the floor as well as trying the patience and good-will of members of your nursing staff (e.g., he is using loud, abusive language and making unreasonable demands on the nursing staff). You, as head nurse, could try to use your authority to force him to change his behavior. Before doing that, however, you may prefer to reason with him without appealing to threats. You point out that his behavior is causing problems for other patients and for the nursing staff. You emphasize that such behavior exhibits a lack of respect for others, that he is (perhaps unwittingly) treating others very badly, that he is not respecting these others as persons. If your patient is able to think rationally and sees that what you are saying about his behavior is true (of course, some patients will be in an emotional condition which makes them incapable of doing this), his own desire to act morally may be sufficient to motivate him to try to change his behavior or at least to make him realize he should do so. In talking with him you have sought a common ground, namely, the fundamental conviction that people are owed respect. Suppose instead you had told him that what he is doing is against God's commandments or the teachings of your rabbi. If you and he happen to be theists, this could be effective. But obviously if he is not, it is unlikely to be.

Consider again the case of the twelve-year-old cancer victim. To be effective in advocating one of the three alternatives, you must appeal to principles the others also accept and show that, consistent with these principles, the alternative you advocate is the option to be preferred. If you appeal to principles that presuppose special theological views not shared by all the others, your effectiveness is diminished.

The basic strategy in moral discussion is to find common ground upon which all parties to the discussion can agree. Since many people today are not religious believers, an ethic that is not detached from its theological context will be less effective than one that is neutral with respect to religious beliefs. We are searching for a moral stance that will be generally applicable, one having the broadest possible use. Nursing is not a religious order. Even those nurses practicing in religiously affiliated hospitals may feel that their action as professionals ought to be broader than that of a particular religious perspective. For this reason, we shall not attempt to resolve any of the moral dilemmas to be considered by appeal to principles that are dependent upon the truth of any theological views. This does not mean, of course, that it would be inappropriate for the reader to supplement the fundamental and general moral stance developed here with specific principles from his or her religious tradition.

Perhaps no other group has paid more careful attention to moral issues in health care than the Roman Catholic Church. Its thinking has greatly affected our laws, institutions, and practices. Some of this reflection is based on theologically neutral moral principles and, therefore, has general applicability. Much of it, however, is embedded in a particular theological perspective, the natural law doctrine. According to natural law theory, the universe is organized in such a way that every kind of thing has a purpose or goal or end *(telos)*. This teleological organization (design, order) must be seen as a product of a divine plan.

Not only are these theological assumptions not shared by the general public, they are quite possibly false. At one time physics and biology appeared to support the doctrine of a teleological organization in the world. Nonetheless, the philosophical support for this view was withdrawn in the seventeenth century's rejection of Aristotle's physics. The firm conviction that there are more adequate alternative accounts of the order found in nature (the operation of natural selection on random mutations) has come about in biology with the acceptance of contemporary evolutionary theory.

With the putative support for the moral theory undermined, the only reasons for accepting it as guidance for one's life appear to be Church authority and tradition. The debate thus changes from one of trying to find good reasons for one's moral judgments to trying to decide by which of the many authorities seeking our allegiance we shall live. But if our moral principles are accepted by appeal to authority, morality can no longer serve a prime function, providing the common ground needed to settle conflicts of interest peaceably.

These general remarks concerning the natural law tradition have been made to support the claim that a moral position that can stand detached from controversial theological assumptions will serve us better than one embedded in such a tradition. We have seen two reasons for this: (a) a basic purpose of morality is to settle conflicts of interest, and to do this effectively common ground must be found; (b) a professional such as a nurse sees himself or herself as nonsectarian, as a member of a group that transcends particular religious, national, or ethnic traditions.

The basic principle which will be provisionally accepted and used as the cornerstone for constructing moral arguments in the pages that follow is the command to treat all persons with the respect owed to rational creatures, a command that has been at the root of most moral thinking in the Western world for thousands of years. As such, it provides us with the common ground required.

The principle of respect for persons, when analyzed and clearly understood, provides us with a standard by which we can assess the moral adequacy of the various principles in the professional codes of ethics. Fortunately, the general thrust of the two professional codes we have examined is in comformity with the principle of respect for persons. The ANA code is especially sensitive to the requirement of treating those in one's care with respect and as rational creatures. The use of "client" (as we shall do henceforth) rather than "patient" to describe the person under nursing care emphasizes the desirability of an active role for the person under treatment and of his or her rights as a rational creature to contribute in a variety of ways to the nurse-client relationship.

Combining the principle of respect for persons with those embodied in the codes, we have some building blocks with which to begin to construct a coherent position.

The Moral Point of View

Most of us have not learned morality by formal instruction but rather by participation in life and by example. We learn morality in much the same way as we learn to speak our native tongue. We find that we hold moral values and principles long before we are able to reflect on them or to decide whether or not to accept them. Some people go through life, firm in their convictions, without ever reflecting on the moral values they have received at their mothers' knees. They remain children of their culture and lack the ability to defend their convictions with rational arguments.

If one's life is sheltered enough and the decisions one makes insignificant enough, customary morality may be sufficient. But such is not the life of the nurse. A modern-day nurse cannot escape the rough and tumble of life or avoid involvement in decisions having far-ranging consequences for the quality of other people's lives. Conventional morality is not adequate. Moral maturity is required. The capacity to reason about beliefs and the sensitivity to see the moral dimensions and implications of her or his actions are essential for the nurse.

Of course, some decisions a nurse makes may have no moral component. That is, they will be nonmoral, involving only technical or factual matters. Yet many of her or his decisions, which may not appear at first to be moral issues, will be seen, upon more careful reflection, to be so. To be able to identify the moral facets of a situation, one must have the maturity to be able to go beyond seeing it simply from a personal perspective or through one's own eyes. One must be able to take the perspective of "everyman" or of any other person, or at least to see it through the eyes of all other involved parties.

There is an important shift in point of view when one moves from a personal perspective to a moral one. Not everyone has the capacity to move beyond the personal. Instead, their range of view is limited to seeing all issues as centered on the self. Nevertheless, those who progress up the ladder of moral maturation are able to take a view that goes beyond the confines of oneself.

The philosopher David Hume (1711–1776) has succinctly described the difference between the personal and the moral points of view.

The notion of morals implies some sentiment common to all mankind, which recommends the same object to general appropation. . . . When a man denominates another his *enemy*, his *rival*, his *antagonist*, his *adversary*, he is understood to speak the language of self-love, and to express sentiments, pecular to himself, and arising from his particular circumstances and situation. But when he bestows on any man the epithets of *vicious* or *odious* or *depraved*, he then speaks another language, and expresses sentiments in which he expects all his audience are to concur with him. He must here . . . depart from his private and particular situation, and must choose a point of view, common to himself with others [Hume, 1957, pp. 113–14].

If one takes this moral point of view, the point of view of "everyman," a view with which he or she expects all others to concur, making an exception of oneself is contradictory. If an action is thought to be wrong for another in a similar situation, it must also be considered wrong for oneself. A person is not making a moral judgment if she or he says that, although there is no significant difference between them, one act is right and the other act is wrong. Unequal or different treatment must be based on a relevant difference, a difference that "everyman" can recognize as such. Moral judgments are not personal whim or bias; they are judgments guided by principles one believes can be shared by all others.

Even young children are quick to sense an injustice if one child gets something desirable and another does not. Suppose, for example, a small girl's brother gets a toy but she does not. She is likely to ask for an account. "Why does he get a toy and I don't?" She expects to have some relevant difference pointed out. Of course, it is a difficult task to determine what differences should really count as differences. Theories of justice are devised to cope with this and other thorny problems. A small child, because of limited experience, may be willing to accept almost any (inadequate) account—for example, "He's bigger than you," "He's a boy, you're a girl," or "You were bad today."

Acceptance of the principle of equal treatment, that all similar cases must be treated similarly, is another mark of morality. If someone is unable or unwilling to do that, such a person is not taking the moral point of view. Treating similar cases similarly entails being willing to accept limits on one's behavior toward others commensurate with those actions one wishes done to oneself. That is, to do to others only what you would want done to you (the Golden Rule). Another way of stating this fundamental mark of morality is to say that an action is a moral action only if one is acting on a principle he or she is willing to have everyone act upon, i.e., is willing to *universalize* the principle of one's action.

To sum up our discussion, two interrelated but distinct marks of morality have been uncovered: (a) the moral point of view entails taking a universal perspective, going beyond a personal view to one that, it is believed, *all* others who reflect on the case or issue and who clearly grasp the relevant factors would come to as well; and (b) the moral point of view entails acceptance of the requirement to universalize one's action, to treat all similar cases similarly, and not to make an exception for oneself.

The Logic of Moral Decision-Making

Happily, many of the moral decisions we must make in life are not difficult, and they pose no problem for us. In many situations we know what we ought to do and we do it. Quite simply, my conscience may tell me what I ought to do, and I may feel no need to go beyond that.

Other situations may be identical with the case above, except for the fact that I find I cannot do what I'm convinced I ought to do. I may be quite certain, for example, that I ought to report to my supervisor a series of medication errors I have seen committed by another nurse. But I cannot bring myself to do it. Perhaps the nurse is a close friend, or perhaps she is someone who could make life very unpleasant for me were she to find out that I was the one who reported the errors to the supervisor. Whatever the reason, I find myself unable to do my duty. I suffer from a *weakness of will*. Even St. Paul in the Epistle to the Romans (7:19) reports that he suffered from this problem: "For I do not do the good I want, but the evil I do not want is what I do."

The problem of weakness of will must be distinguished from other obstacles to doing the right thing. In contrast to the other hazards on the path to doing one's duty that we shall consider, weakness of will does not stem from a lack of relevant factual or moral knowledge or a conflict among moral principles themselves. The conflict that arises when one knows what ought to be done but fails to do it is not a conflict *within* morality. It is a struggle within oneself that is not resolved by clearer thinking but by determined effort. In cases of weakness of will or temptation, we *know* what our duty is, but for a variety of reasons (laziness, greed, selfishness, or timidity) we just cannot bring ourselves to do it.

An appeal to conscience may be an entirely satisfactory way to decide what to do in many situations. The more complex the issue, however, the more likely it is that an appeal to conscience will prove ineffectual. Either your conscience will have nothing to tell you about the issue or it will seem to pull you in different directions. For example, suppose you are caring for an elderly person whose physician and family have decided not to inform her of a very bleak prognosis. You doubt the wisdom of this decision. She asks you very pointedly about the results of the series of tests she has undergone. You feel very strongly about the duty of a nurse to be open and forthright with her or his clients. Yet you also feel very strongly that you have a duty to be part of the team, to work in concert with others for a coherent course of treatment. In cases such as this, one needs a more refined instrument than conscience.

An appeal to conscience is also ineffective as a way of persuading others of the rightness or wrongness of a particular moral judgment. The verdicts of my conscience are confined to my actions, just as the verdicts of your conscience are confined to yours. My conscience cannot tell you what you ought or ought not to do. If my conscience tells me one thing and yours another, we have no way to resolve our differences. Although we cannot both be right, neither can admit to being wrong, nor can either be justified in going against his or her own conscience as a way to resolve the conflict. This is a serious limitation, since one of the main purposes of engaging in moral discussion is to settle conflicts of interest. You want to be in a position to be able to persuade me, just as I want to be in a position to persuade you. These considerations also lead us to the conclusion that we must go beyond appeals to conscience.

Suppose you have made a moral decision and you are called upon to explain your action. We have seen that saying "I followed my conscience" is a very weak response. If you did what you thought was right, what you would try to do in offering a satisfactory response would be to show why it was right by giving reasons that others would also find persuasive. As we saw before, when taking the moral point of view, one is taking a position one believes will also be taken by all others who think about the issue in an unbiased and clear way.

In giving reasons for your actions you could appeal to your *duties as a nurse*. For example, you could point to one of the duties outlined in the ANA *Code for Nurses*. Duties often arise from the *role* we play, whether it be professional, familial, or societal. Or you could point to a particular *obligation* you incurred by a previous commitment; for example, you made a promise you are obliged to keep. Or finally, you could appeal to some *moral rule* that you feel is binding and applicable in the case at hand. For example, you may appeal to the moral rule to tell the truth or the rule to treat others with the respect owed to persons. Appeal to any one or any combination of moral directives— (a) the duties one has as a nurse (arising from one's role), (b) the particular obligations one has incurred, (c) general moral rules—can form the basis of one's account of his or her actions as a moral agent.

As long as only one duty, obligation, or moral rule applies, one's concern must be with interpreting it and determining how it applies in the case at hand. For example, if the only moral rule, duty, or obligation applicable to your situation is your professional duty to safeguard your client's right to privacy, you can appeal to the second principle of the ANA nursing code. You know what action guide to follow: you must judiciously protect information of a confidential nature. Application requires determining just what course of action optimally satisfies this moral directive. Practical knowledge and experience must supplement the moral directive in making this determination. For example, if you know that, in your present context, putting the information on the client's chart is tantamount to making it public, you may have to act differently than you would if you were in a situation in which you could count on the client's chart being held in strict confidence (that is, it will not go beyond the circle of the health team). Practical knowledge and experience are also necessary to determine whether what is told to one in confidence is in fact true. It may not be true at all but rather a way of calling for help or gaining attention. Obviously, different circumstances affect how one should apply the moral directive to keep confidences. No formula can be provided for making these determinations. Effective moral decision-making requires the psychological sensitivity that comes from living and from experience with persons in all sorts of situations. It also requires knowledge of the institutions within which one functions.

Moral decision-making may sound extremely complex and appear to be something a busy and over-worked nurse would have little time or energy for. Nevertheless, we have not yet considered the even more complex and important cases that the nurse must confront, *moral dilemmas.* A person is faced with a moral dilemma when several duties, obligations, or moral rules are applicable to the situation but when following one or more of these precludes following any of the others. Several of the cases we have considered have the form of the moral dilemma. In the case of the twelve-year-old cancer victim, we saw that following the duty to alleviate suffering (stopping treatment and increasing the narcotic dosage) conflicts with the duty to conserve life (increasing the dosage could hasten death), and following the duty to conserve life (continuing modest treatment and not increasing the narcotic dosage) obviously conflicts with the duty to alleviate suffering.

In the case just described, two role-related duties are in conflict. Many other possible combinations of conflicting directives are possible. A role-related duty can be in conflict with a particular obligation one has incurred or with a moral rule. Two moral rules can conflict.

Any time more than one role-related duty, obligation, or moral rule applies to a particular situation, the possibility of conflict is there.

Let us consider one more case of conflict, a conflict of the rule-related duty to "hold in confidence all personal information entrusted to" the nurse and the moral rule to tell the truth. Suppose that in the course of a conversation with a client, he divulges personal information about himself which is clearly meant to remain confidential. He tells you that he has given up all hope of recovering sufficiently to be able to return home. He especially does not want his family to know this because he feels they will see his giving up hope as an indication that he does not want to get well. And that would make them sad. A few days later, a member of his family asks you if he has ever talked to you about his hopes and expectations and when he thinks he will be strong enough to come home. If you do not engage in deception (either by telling a falsehood or by skillfully evading the question so as to lead the questioner to conclude that you do not know your client's feelings on this issue) you will not have succeeded in fully keeping the confidence. One or the other directive (keeping the confidence or telling the truth) cannot be followed. By deciding in favor of one you decide against the other.

Obviously, what we would like to have when confronted with moral dilemmas in a nonarbitrary way to determine which rule to follow and which to violate. *If* we could demonstrate that certain directives always take priority over others—e.g., that the duty to keep confidences takes priority over the rule to tell the truth, or that role-related duties take priority over other obligations or moral rules, then we would have a clear, rational decision procedure for making these judgments. If you test it (by thinking of a variety of cases in which the two duties conflict), you will probably find that in some cases you will feel the duty to keep confidences should take priority, but in other cases the duty to tell the truth should. So the specific suggestion for resolving this dilemma is unacceptable. Yet the general strategy suggested is promising. The way out of these moral dilemmas is to find some way to order the relevant directives. For example, we may be able to find some more basic principle which we can appeal to in conflict situations. Suppose, for purposes of illustration, we were to determine that the following moral principle was a more basic one: act so as to produce the greatest balance of good over evil for all people affected by your action. We could then appeal to this principle as a way to resolve the conflict between the duties of confidentiality and truth-telling. The way to decide which duty has priority would be to determine what the consequences will be for each alternative. The alternative to choose is the one that is likely to produce the best consequences—i.e., the greatest balance of good over evil for all persons.

The problem of ordering the duties and moral principles is one of the most difficult ones with which ethical theorists struggle. There is no consensus as to which principles or duties are more basic than others. Since ethical theorists have been unable to resolve this issue, it would be foolhardy for us to attempt to resolve it in a book on applied ethics. What we can do, however, is to see that some ways of ordering the moral directives are superior to others. To do this we will have to consider several ethical theories.

Before we focus on the question of the ordering of our moral directives, it will be instructive to take up the issue of moral disagreements. On the basis of what we now know about the logic of moral reasoning, we can see the various points at which disagreement is possible. One of the most important skills one can learn in order to engage in moral discussion effectively is to be able to determine the exact point in the reasoning process at which the disagreement arises.

Moral Disagreements

We have all had experiences in which we strongly disagreed with another person about a particular issue, only to discover later that our disagreement was based on a misunderstanding. Had we been clearer about what each of us was asserting, we would have avoided the misunderstanding. Conversely, we may have felt we were in full agreement with someone, only to discover later that we had fundamental differences. Clarity requires that we consider the various points at which disagreement can occur and work out a check list to be used to pinpoint the problem in particular disagreements.

The framework for this discussion is already in place, since we developed the logic of moral decision-making in the previous section. We have seen that reasoning leading to moral decisions includes appeals to one or more moral rules, duties, or obligations, as well as assertions or tacit assumptions about facts, i.e., about what is the case. As we shall see, in beginning with the simpler cases and moving to the more complex, there are several different points at which disagreement can occur.

First consider a case in which only one moral principle is involved. For purposes of illustration, let us take the rule of truth-telling. Suppose a nurse is asked to administer a placebo (a "sugar pill" or other inert compound given for its suggestive effect). His client asks him what it is he is giving her. He answers that it is an injection that should ease her pain. Later he tells another nurse what he did and said. She disagrees with him in his contention that his action was morally acceptable behavior.

Let us try to determine more specifically what the disagreement might be. If the disagreement is over the moral rule to tell the truth, there are two very different points at which disagreement can arise. (A) Disagreement concerning the validity of the principle or rule: One party to the disagreement may hold that we have a general duty to tell the truth. The other may hold that there is no such duty. For example, someone could argue that what must be done in each situation is that action which will produce the greatest overall good. Truth-telling is a duty only in cases in which telling the truth produces the most general good. So in cases such as this one in which failure to tell the truth (let us suppose) results in greater good (the client's pain is decreased without having to use drugs that may have deleterious side effects), the truth-telling rule lacks validity. (B) Disagreement concerning the applicability of the principle or rule: Both parties to the dispute may agree on the validity of the truth-telling principle. Yet one may argue, contrary to the other, that the principle does not apply to the case at hand. The issue here is not (so the argument might go) one of failing to tell the truth or telling a lie. Given the placebo effect (the fact that expecting relief can bring it about), the placebo that was administered is likely to ease her pain. So, contrary to first appearances, nothing false was said. The principle concerning truth-telling does not bear on the decision to administer a placebo in this case. On the other hand, the other party to the dispute may see this as clearly a truth-telling issue. He or she may argue that there is a natural presumption that an injection would contain an active ingredient. Administering the injection and saying it will ease the pain trades on this presumption. Done as it was, the intention was to deceive the client. So (the argument continues) the question of giving this client a placebo in the manner described is inescapably a truth-telling matter. Finally, if the validity of the truth-telling principle is not questioned, it is applicable in this case; therefore we must conclude that the action is wrong.

At this point we need not go into any more detail on all the various responses that could be made to these arguments. (The issue will be examined with great care in Chapter 5). For our present purposes, however, it is instructive to consider one retort to the final argument just discussed. Someone might say that he or she agrees that the case of administering the placebo is a case to which the truth-telling principle applies. Yet he or she refuses to conclude that the action is wrong because it is asserted that another duty also has bearing on the case and this other duty takes priority over the truth-telling requirement. Suppose this other duty is the nurse's duty to cooperate and assist in administering the course of treatment best designed to bring about recovery.

This possible retort to the argument concluding that giving the placebo was morally objectionable uncovers two additional sources of disagreement. (C) Disagreement concerning either the validity or applicability of other principles, duties, or obligations: For each of these we repeat the questions asked in (A) and (B) above. (D) Disagreement concerning the proper ordering of the principles (rules, obligation, duties): In the retort given, the claim was made that the duty to cooperate in the treatment plan took precedence over the requirement to tell the truth. Clearly someone could disagree with this ordering, saying that the duty to tell the truth is the more stringent duty. The case of the twelve-year-old cancer patient discussed earlier is another example of disagreements arising from differing views as to the proper ordering of the relevant moral duties (those of alleviating suffering, promoting health, conserving life).

In sum, disagreements about moral principles can be about their validity, their applicability to the case at hand, and to their proper ordering or ranking. Progress on resolving these conflicts requires being clear as to which of these (whether any or all) is the source of the disagreement.

If the disagreement does not lie in any of these points, (E) the disagreement must be in the factual or empirical (the IS) as opposed to the normative (the OUGHT) components of the argument. Imagine that we have come to a common position on the normative questions, yet we still disagree about the placebo case. We must then have a different view of the facts of the case. Upon examination let us say that we discover the real reason for our inability to agree on the case is that one of us is inclined to disagree with the assumptions that administering the placebo is the best way to help the client, while the other believes it is the medically indicated course (the course of treatment with the best prospects for success). Resolution of this difference requires a reconsideration of nonmoral issues, including principles of psychology, the placebo effect, alternative modes of treatment, and so on—the technical problems that form part of the core of a medical or nursing curriculum.

We shall focus on the disagreements that arise concerning moral principles A through D. Still, this emphasis should not be construed as suggesting that factual disagreements are readily resolvable. It may be extremely difficult to determine what the consequences of a course of action will be—to take just one instance of factual knowledge. For example, will telling the truth to this client with the dismal prognosis be devastating and undermine her will to live? Or will it, in some ways, be a relief (with the days and nights of uneasiness and uncertainty being replaced by saying "good-byes" and putting her affairs in order)? We may strongly disagree on what, in fact, would occur. The facts can also be incredibly complex, such as, for example, trying to determine whether a person is suffering from a rare disease that has many symptoms in common with other diseases.

Clearly, resolving factual differences may be difficult. Determining what the facts are may require all the skill and knowledge of the psychiatrist, medical and nurse researcher, historian, political scientist, and so on. All of the scientific procedures devised to discover the truth and to accurately express it can be used to attempt to resolve these issues. Professional training gives one the tools to cope with these issues. How to resolve differences over the nonfactual component of moral reasoning is the concern in this book.

There is no guarantee that isolating and focusing upon the points of disagreement will result in agreement. It *will* result in better understanding and in debates with others that are to the point. Whether you feel agreement will result frequently or only rarely will depend upon your own experience and also upon whether you are generally an optimist or a pessimist. Some people are very pessimistic about achieving any kind of agreement on normative issues. For some, their pessimism is based on a thesis that normative ethical principles are *simply* products of the culture, social class, or profession out of which they arise. So (they contend) one certainly cannot expect agreement among people from different professions or different cultural groups— even if agreement were attainable within such groups.

Is it reasonable for us to cast our lot with the pessimists? The difficulty we have in trying to achieve agreement on these issues seems to support doing so. Yet it does not follow from the mere fact that something is difficult that it cannot be done. Also from the fact that ethical principles are the products of our social institutions it does not follow that they are *no more than* that—i.e., that their validity cannot extend beyond the members of the group of genesis or adoption. Science also is a product of certain cultural developments, arising in some cultures and not in others, being accepted in some and rejected in others. Yet we do not conclude that because science is a product of particular cultures and is rejected by many that it would not be possible for all rational persons—whatever their social class, culture, or profession—to agree about certain fundamental scientific principles as well as certain specific explanations of natural phenomena. The hope that propels scientific investigation is one that can also reasonably propel ethical investigation.

Now we turn to the final section of Chapter 1, a discussion of some of the suggestions ethical theorists have given concerning the ordering of basic moral principles and duties.

Some Basic Moral Principles

A primary concern of ethical theorists is to determine the relationships between and among the various moral rules, duties, and obligations that are appealed to in making moral judgments about particular cases. They ask whether these many principles can be brought together into a unified theory.

Earlier we mentioned that theories are designed to assist us in conflict-of-duty situations by helping us to give a priority ordering to the principles. Obviously, the ideal theory for purposes of resolving these conflicts and for deciding moral issues in the most rational and least arbitrary way would be a theory that had *one* ultimate principle that underlies and explains all the rest.

Suppose that we were to accept the following as the one ultimate principle: we ought to do those actions that produce the greatest balance of happiness (pleasure) over unhappiness (pain) for all affected parties. Suppose that this principle is seen to be the final court of appeal. Consider, then, the case discussed earlier of the child with cancer. What to do in this case—which of the three alternatives (increase the narcotic dosage, continue modest treatment without increasing the narcotic dosage, engage in another surgical procedure) to give priority to—would be answered by determining which alternative would, in fact, produce the greatest total good, taking into account the interests of all involved persons. The alternative that would result in the greatest overall good is the one we ought to follow.

Ethical theorists who maintain that the ultimate principle is one having to do with best consequences for all concerned (as in the above illustration) are *utilitarians*. The ultimate principle—which can be stated in a variety of ways—is called the *principle of utility* (Pr.U.). The theories of two nineteenth-century British philosophers, Jeremy Bentham (1748–1832) and John Stuart Mill (1806–1873), have come to be spoken of as "classical utilitarianism." Mill stated that the principle of utility "holds that actions are right in proportion as they tend to promote happiness; wrong as they tend to promote the reverse of happiness" (Mill, 1957, p. 10).

Over the years, the utilitarian theory has come to be presented in two major forms—*act-utilitarianism* and *rule-utilitarianism*. The crucial difference between these two forms is the status of rules. For act-utilitarianism, rules are, at most, generalizations we can make from past experience. For example, in general, experience has revealed that truth-telling leads to the best consequences. Rules are no more than *rules of thumb*, such as the rule in football to punt on fourth down. One must not slavishly follow a rule if, in one's particular situation, better consequences for all can be served by disregarding the rule. In each situation, one must determine which of the possible alternative courses of action is the most beneficial, having taken into account the interests of all affected persons. The right action is the one that will produce the greatest benefit. Act-utilitarianism can be diagrammed as follows: Pr.U. → Action.

The act-utilitarian formulation allows for great flexibility. One is not bound by rules when adherence to them would fail to maximize the good. One is free to apply the "greatest good for the greatest number principle" in each situation. Because the one principle is applied to each situation, this view is sometimes called situation ethics.

Unfortunately, utilitarianism in this simple formulation appears not to be adequate. It condones—even requires—actions which are quite reprehensible. For example, suppose a client, on her deathbed, has asked you to tell her children who are unable to be with her about the incredible suffering she had to endure at the end and how she became convinced (as you are) that the medical treatment she was given was a mistake. You agree to do so. Later you (correctly) see that greater good could be served by not telling them. In gratitude to the hospital for the care they believe it gave their mother while they unavoidably were away, they wish to make a donation toward the purchase of badly needed equipment—something they would not do if you kept your promise. Using the act-utilitarian theory we must conclude that it is right to break your promise. The theory does not give any special weight to previous commitments. It is simply *forward looking*. Only when keeping commitments, such as promises, contributes to future good are they to be honored.

Beside not doing justice to our obligations such as promise-keeping, the theory does not account for our sense of individual justice. Suppose we are doing research on clients' responses to different ways nurses could administer a particular treatment. We know that one way has proved effective, but it is quite costly and time consuming. We experiment with other less costly and less time-consuming modes of care, hoping to find a better alternative. Since we know none of our clients would be willing to forego the proven treatment in favor of one which, in fact, is likely to be much less effective, we do not inform them of the standard treatment. Now suppose that this will not have any negative legal ramifications and that the experimental design will give us the vital information in the most-efficient and timely fashion. The benefits will quite clearly outweigh the costs which must be borne by a few clients. Of course, this study—although justifiable according to act-utilitarianism—is morally objectionable. It runs roughshod over the clients' rights; it treats them as means for the advancement of society's interests. This example reveals that the act-utilitarian theory lacks an adequate theory of justice.

The more-complex form of utilitarianism—rule-utilitarianism—has been developed in part as a way to meet the criticisms directed against act-utilitarianism. Rule-utilitarianism adds an intermediate step between the basic principle of utility and the decision concerning what action to perform. The intermediate step is a set of rules which have passed the utility test. The rules that come to play a central role are determined by asking which rules will promote the greatest general good for everyone.

The question is not which *action* has the greatest utility, but which *rule* has. The principle of utility comes in, normally at least, not in determining what particular action to perform (this is normally determined by the rules), but in determining what the rules shall be. Rules must be selected, maintained, revised, and replaced on the basis of their utility and not on any other basis. The principle of utility is still the ultimate standard, but it is to be appealed to at the level of rules rather than at the level of particular judgments [Frankena, 1973, p. 39].

Rule-utilitarianism can be diagrammed as follows:

Pr.U. → Rules → Actions.

Rule-utilitarianism maintains that we are better off if we have a set of rules that are always observed. For example, a rule-utilitarian might argue that the greatest general good is served if health care facilities or teams were to adopt a set of rules to guide them in individual decisions. These rules would be selected and, when necessary, revised by running the utility test on them. Examples of rules that health teams—in many contemporary settings—would likely find serve utility best would be: (a) tell the truth unless your client requests that you not do so or if doing so would *undoubtedly* cause him or her great harm; (b) provide all necessary care for the terminally ill unless your client requests that no heroic efforts be made; (c) obtain informed consent prior to all but emergency procedures.

Rule-utilitarianism does appear to be a more satisfactory view than act-utilitarianism. It does not condone certain obviously wrong actions, as is the case (as we have seen) for at least the simplist form of act-utilitarianism. Yet, upon reflection, you may find that it too is not entirely adequate, that it too fails to capture all that we want to be saying in making moral judgments. We can quite readily imagine contexts or cultures in which adopting a rule such as rule *c* above concerning informed consent would not serve the greatest general good. Despite this, however, you may feel that it would be wrong to engage in treatments on people's bodies without their informed consent. You might be inclined to say that informed consent is a requirement for nonemergency intervention even if it does not produce the greatest general good.

If you are inclined to reason in this way, it is because you feel the force of the fundamental moral principle of the Hebrew-Christian tradition: it is impermissible to fail to treat all human beings as rational creatures. Intervention without consent fails to respect the other's rationality, autonomy, and right to self-determination. As we saw earlier (see the Hebrew-Christian Moral Tradition above), Immanuel Kant's ethical theory takes this to be (one form of) the fundamental principle of morality.

Kant argued that consequences do not make an action right or wrong. The morally relevant factor is the principle upon which we act. We must act out of respect for the moral law, which is acting in accordance with what we have called the moral point of view (the willingness to universalize one's actions) and the fundamental Hebrew-Christian principle (respect for persons). Only those actions which are in conformity with these requirements—which Kant considers to be two forms of the Categorical Imperative—are morally acceptable.

Kant's view introduces a necessary corrective to utilitarianism. It protects the individual against claims that his or her life, freedom, rights, or dignity must be sacrificed to increase the general happiness.

Less persuasive is Kant's claim that consideration of consequences is not only irrelevant but even an inappropriate consideration when making moral judgments. Morality has been created to settle conflicts of interests in ways that will promote the fullest expression of these interests compatible with a like expression for others. It follows that morality must not only do what Kant wants it to do (protect individual autonomy and dignity) but also what utilitarians want it to do (advance the general good). Morality has a *protective* function but also a *promotive* function. An adequate theory must account for both and provide some means for balancing these two concerns.

Our discussion leads us to the conclusion that two interrelated principles form the core of an acceptable view: the Kantian respect for persons principle and a basic principle presupposed by utilitarian theories, the *principle of beneficence*—a principle which states that we ought to do good to and for anyone and to prevent or avoid doing harm to anyone.

If we did not have this more basic obligation [the principle of beneficence], we could have no duty to try to realize the greatest balance of good over evil. In fact, the principle of utility represents a compromise with the ideal. The ideal is to do only good and not to do any harm. . . . But this is often impossible, and then we seem forced to try to bring about the best possible balance of good over evil. If this is so, then the principle of utility presupposes a more basic principle—that of producing good as such and preventing evil. We have a prima facie obligation to maximize the balance of good over evil only if we have a *prior* prima facie obligation to do good and prevent harm [Frankena, 1973, p. 45].

On the basis of the criticisms we have leveled against utilitarianism and the fact that the principle of utility is not basic but presupposes a more basic principle (the principle of beneficence), we conclude that utilitarianism does not offer an adequate foundation for our discussion of moral issues in nursing. Instead we adopt the Kantian principle of respect for persons as our most fundamental principle.

One of the obvious ways we show respect for persons is by *refraining* from harming them or refraining from inflicting evil upon them. This is one of four elements as well of the principle of beneficence, our penultimate principle. A second element of the principle of beneficence is that we ought to *prevent* evil or harm. Third, we ought to *remove* evil. Fourth, we ought to do or *promote* good.

Of these four elements, a *presumption* can be made that the first takes precedence over (i.e., is more stringent than) the second, the second over the third, and the third over the fourth (cf. Frankena, 1973, p. 47). Were we to claim that in a particular case our duty to do one of the higher ranked duties (e.g., removing evil) should take precedence over a lower ranked one (e.g., refraining from harming another), the burden of proof falls on us, and we must be prepared to give weighty reasons. In short, the ordering of these principles is not absolute, but any departures from the ordering are to be made with great reluctance and with very good reason.

This ordering of principles is consistent with the ancient medical ethics dictum, "Above all else, do no harm." It is also consistent with the Pauline principle that evil is not to be done that good may come of it.

Far more work on fundamentals would be necessary before we could be confident that we had uncovered not only the basic principles of morality but also the proper ordering of them. Ethical theorists dedicate their lives to this pursuit. The basic principles and ordering we have proposed should be seen as having heuristic value as well as having support from several honorable traditions and from our own reflection. We do not begin on the bedrock of certainty, but neither is our starting point arbitrary.

2

The Role of the Nurse

We saw in Chapter 1 that one of the sources of our moral directives is our role, whether it be professional, familial, or societal. In this chapter we shall examine the changing and expanding role of the nurse and see how these changes influence moral problems in nursing. The changes that have occurred and are occurring make it especially difficult to be clear about the nurse's role-related duties. At times such as these we get very little guidance from tradition and custom—for they, too, are being questioned. Nevertheless, a look at the traditional model of the nurse can help us understand how it is that we have come to be in the present state of flux.

Until recently nurses have been viewed (by the public and nurses themselves) as dependent functionaries, acting under the direction and supervision of physicians. In a recent study of hospitalized patients, those queried mentioned the following as nursing functions: taking doctors' orders, giving medications, serving meals, giving shots, and providing bedpans (Beletz, 1974). The nurse's role has frequently been viewed as being analogous to that of the traditional wife and mother in a household.

When the first American schools of nursing were established the family was the institutional model for the operation of hospitals. All policies and procedures formulated to guide management of the "household" were designed to look out for the overall interests of the institution. . . . The role of [nurses] was very early conceived as that of caring for the "hospital family" . . . Like mothers in a household, nurses were responsible for meeting the needs of all members of the hospital family—from patients to physicians [Ashley, 1977, p. 17].

The concept of the nurse as "surrogate mother" with the physician as (traditional) husband and father (i.e., as head of the household) and client as child has not only been widely held in the past, it continues to be held by many today.

A related model of the nurse—one that stresses even more than the surrogate mother model the nurse's dependency relationship to the physician—is that of "handmaiden of the physician" (female servant or attendant). The nurse is seen as the physician's personal assistant, who can provide technical and humane services which nurture the client. The nurse is not a decision-maker nor one to initiate treatment. She (or he) lacks the knowledge for that. She is able only to implement the physician's decisions.

With these two as the dominant models of nursing in early and mid-twentieth century, it is not surprising that 97 percent of nurses are women (Navarro, 1975, p. 400). This, despite the fact that in earlier times men were much more prominent in the nursing profession. "Historically nursing has been done by men since the Crusades in both the religious and the secular contexts. Even in the United States a large percentage of nursing services was performed by men in the early part of the 19th century" (Aroskar, 1980, p. 21).

These days it is frequently argued—for example, by Joann Ashley in *Hospitals, Paternalism, and the Role of the Nurse* and by Mila Ann Aroskar in the article just cited—that nursing has come to be regarded as a feminine (passive, submissive) role because most nurses are women, and in a male-dominated, sexist society such as ours, women are seen as (and see themselves as) dependent and subservient. As Robert Baker has pointed out, however, another possible way to account for the disproportionate number of females in nursing is that they "have been channeled into nursing because the profession, *by its very nature*, requires its members to play a dependent and subservient role (i.e., the traditional female role in a sexist society)" [Baker, 1980, pp. 42–43].

Our task is not that of constructing the most-adequate historical account of the fact that nursing in the mid-twentieth century is regarded as a feminine role. What is important for our purposes is to determine whether nursing, by its very nature, requires its members to play a dependent and subservient role. The moral duties one has as a "dependent professional" (the title of an editorial by Rozella Schlotfeldt, 1976) are quite different from those one has as an autonomous professional. The ANA *Code for Nurses* is premised on the notion of the nurse as an autonomous professional and on the concept of the nurse as client advocate. One of the sharpest contrasts between it and the (earlier) *International Code of Nursing Ethics* is that of the view of the nurse presupposed by the codes. The International Code has not moved far from the traditional notion of dependency upon the physician. Whereas the ANA code entails that the nurse's primary duty is to the client, the International Code entails that her or his fundamental allegiance is to the physician. The contrast is most clearly evident by comparing clause three of the ANA code with clauses seven and eight of the International Code. (See the codes and discussion of them in Chapter 1.)

There are several reasons why many nurses and others who are interested in the well-being of the nursing profession favor a model of nursing such as that of client advocate, and who find the traditional surrogate mother and handmaiden of the physician models inadequate and objectionable. Most of these reasons (some of which we shall discuss below) are nonmoral reasons (i.e., they are concerned with factors such as efficiency of care, political power, and so on). Yet they are relevant to our task because (as we have seen) the role-related duties a nurse has are contingent upon the role which has been adopted. Let us consider the variety of reasons the traditional models have lost favor with many.

A. The sex-role stereotyping with which these models are linked has been challenged by the women's liberation (feminist) movement. We have all seen that if we take away the blind, unthinking adherence to gender or sex-role stereotypes and eliminate the coercive practices that make it difficult for members of either sex to step beyond the cultural definitions of male and female work, many women are no longer content to play the submissive, passive role. We see that many more women than in the past are going into fields previously considered as male domains. But even those going into the traditional female occupations have changed. Students in baccalaureate nursing programs today appear to be less inclined to fall into a submissive role than did students ten or more years ago [Davis, 1969; DeLora and Moses, 1969].

B. Our concept of the proper roles of family members has changed. Many factors have produced this change in outlook: the breakdown of sex-role stereotypes (just discussed), changing economic circumstances (high percentages of two-income family units), changing birth rates (fewer children per couple), experimentation with alternative family structures (for example, a family unit headed by two females rather than a husband and a wife), and the breakdown of an increasingly large number of marriages, resulting in single-parent family units. With all these changes in the basic family model, it no longer seems obvious that other institutions need be patterned after the traditional model. Other models with rather different implications for the role of the nurse can now be considered. Experience has demonstrated that the mother's and the wife's role can be quite different from the traditional conception. So, too, can roles (e.g., nursing) that have been based on the models of mother and wife.

C. Technological advances in the care of the sick have also affected both the practice and the conception of the role of the nurse. Especially in hospital care, changing technology has resulted in extending the responsibility of nurses. Often for very practical reasons, nurses have been delegated authority to carry out duties initially assigned only to physicians. An example from one area of nursing is representative of a rather common phenomenon.

Careful research into the nurse's role in the coronary care unit indicates that it came about primarily as a result of default, dictate, *and* exigency, and not from careful analysis of the role by the nursing profession. Doctors staffed one of the original coronary care units that later served as the prototype of many other units, until they rebelled against the boredom and constant vigilance; then nurses, who are believed somehow different in temperament so that they really understand boring vigils, were assigned to replace the doctors. When it became obvious that the nurse's vigilance was not enough in the coronary care unit, it was conveniently reasoned that the same nurses, who throughout history were thought to be capable only of observing and reporting, could now not only detect a potentially fatal arrhythmia, but were capable also of terminating it with a complex electronic device—capable, that is, only in the event the physician did not arrive in the critical first two minutes [Berwind, 1975, p. 89].

D. The changing age distribution of the population has resulted in a greater need for the kinds of services nursing best provides. The number of people in the postretirement age group is rapidly increasing. People of advanced age are more likely than others to need the nurture, the care, the emotional support, the long-term monitoring, and the teaching necessary to cope with diminished capacities that nurses are well-suited to provide. The aged suffering from chronic illness need *care* and sustenance rather than *cure*. Often in these cases, the highly technical and interventionist skills of the physician are, in fact, ancillary to the caring functions of the nurse.

Of course, in reality the power has usually remained in the hands of the physician, whose position is securely buttressed by the law and tradition. But the physician's position as perpetual "captain of the team" appears to square with neither the way services are actually provided today nor efficiency in their delivery. The exalted position of physicians appears to have no basis other than their desire to hold on to a position of power and prestige. Those concerned with efficiency of health care delivery, cost-cutting, as well as the prestige and professional standing of nurses argue for an increasingly active and autonomous role for nurses in cases in which care rather than cure is the primary need.

No longer is the physician automatically viewed as the captain of the team and the source of all information about patients' needs. There are well over 200 categories of health workers, and a number of them increasingly view themselves as professionals whose education and expertise enable them to make judgments and decisions in a specific area of health care. Medical care is an aspect of health care, but so are nursing care, special therapies, and others [Sward, 1980, p. 9].

A case for the primacy of nursing care can be made not only for an increasing number of aged who are chronically ill but also for those (of any age) recognized as incurable. Such people are beyond the help of physicians but clearly are not beyond the help of nurses.

By their declaration of incurability physicians have admitted that nothing can be done to ameliorate sickness. But if death is inevitable, pain and incapacity need not be, and the tasks and roles that they set for themselves help incurable patients satisfy their own, often internal, task-role expectations as much as they possibly can. The role of the nurse is to care for the sick in their sickness, even when cure is impossible [Baker, 1980, p. 45].

An example of nursing care as primary, with physician's care as ancillary, is the hospice movement, one of which is St. Christopher's.

St. Christopher's is a nursing facility for the incurably ill directed by Cicely Saunders—a nurse who, in order to have her theories of nursing the incurably ill listened to, had to qualify as a physician. At St. Christopher's, care of the sick is primary; disease *per se* is untreated, and physicians are indeed ancillary to nurses [Baker, 1980, p. 45].

(The topic of nursing and hospices will be treated in Chapter 4, part 4, "Nursing and the Dying Patient.")

These (A–D) and undoubtedly other factors have contributed to the dissatisfaction with the traditional conceptions of the nurse's role and the search for a more appropriate one. All seem to agree on at least one feature of an appropriate model, namely, that the nurse must be viewed as more than a dependent functionary. She or he may quite appropriately work at times under a physician. But that is not the defining characteristic of the profession.

A small number of nurses (nurse practitioners—about 13,000 of the 1.4 million licensed nurses) have extended the role of the nurse by adding to their functions many that traditionally have been done by physicians. They take clients' health histories, make referrals to physicians, perform diagnostic procedures, make initial house calls to assess a client's condition, initiate treatment in cardiac arrest, prescribe medications for certain conditions, and so on. All this is done under the supervision of a physician, but the nurse practitioner has considerable latitude. The greater responsibility and decision-making authority is what distinguishes the practitioner from the traditional nurse as "handmaiden of the physician." Yet she or he remains "an extension of the physician's hands."

There are two rather different, yet *not* necessarily incompatible, ways the search for a more adequate role has taken. On the one hand, as we saw earlier, the nurse's role can be *distinguished from* that of the physician. Whereas the physician's function is (roughly speaking) to cure, the nurse's is to care (the hospice movement is an example). On the other hand, as we have just seen with the nurse practitioner (which is modeled after, and very similar to, the physician's assistant program), the nurse's role can be seen as *identical with* a segment of the physician's traditional responsibilities.

The role of the nurse is expanding in both of these ways: traditional nursing *care* functions have increased in importance (for reasons already discussed), while the traditional function of assisting a physician has greatly gained in scope. An adequate understanding of the nurse's role must encompass both of these developments. Frequently, however, one of these dimensions of the expanding role is stressed at the expense of the other.

When similarities between nursing and medicine are emphasized, the role of the nurse can be expanded into those (a) areas and (b) functions which suffer as a result of the uneven distribution of, and lack of, general practitioners. Examples of (a) are the nurse practitioners with organizations such as the National Health Service who frequently are the only full-time health professional in a county which has no physician. Examples of (b) are nurse practitioners who perform the basic diagnostic functions of the general practitioner in order to admit clients into the health care network. That is, the nurse performs the "gate-keeping" function, determining who needs the services of the various professionals within the health care facility. It seems likely that nursing will continue to expand in these ways and that the nurse practitioner—many of whom may go into private practice—will play an ever-increasing role in the delivery of health care. One of many recent developments in which we can see this occurring is in the design of health maintenance organizations (HMOs). "The enactment of federal legislation to encourage development of health maintenance organizations makes clarification of the role of nurse practitioner a high priority. . . . As health maintenance organizations grow—and in other frameworks as well—the nurse practitioner will be a key member of the health team" [Roemer, 1975, p. 49].

These are important developments and ones that promise greater efficiency and better use of personnel resources than will be the case if we continue to insist that these services remain in the sphere of the physician. The developments are also attractive to many nurses, who yearn for greater responsibility and opportunity. It would be a mistake to consider the nurse practitioner as the paradigm for the nurse of the future, however. Nursing is much broader than this. The most-serious loss with such a concept of nursing would be the failure to capture the quality that sets nursing apart from the other health professions, namely, a special kind of client *care*.

We have compared the curative function of the physician with the care or nurturing function of the nurse. It is in this contrast with physicians that we touch the core of nursing, the feature that cannot be absent if nursing is present. The distinction between physician cure and nursing care developed earlier is most vividly captured by the image of the physician stopping momentarily by the bedside to see how the treatment plan is progressing, while the nurse is at the bedside 24 hours a day providing care, comfort, and compassion. The most-vital human dimension of health care—a dimension which increases in importance as our society becomes increasingly domi-nated by technology—is what the nurse *qua* nurse has to offer. "In a society of machines, in institutions of healing run by machines, the nurse has a vital part to play in preserving the human aspects of patient care" [Wilson, 1974, p. 414].

Examination of the nurse's role reveals that its unique contribution to client care is maintaining the human element in what would otherwise become cold, uncaring, and depersonalized treatment. The nurse's role is, at its fundamental level, a moral one, one of insuring the dignity and autonomy of the client in need. The fundamental question concerning the nurse's role is what conception of the nurse will likely result in the most-effective and efficient exercising of this primary nursing responsibility to ensure humane, dignified care.

Rather than seeing oneself as a mother surrogate or as an extension of the physician, clearly a far better model for achieving the primary nursing care objective is that of the client's advocate. On this view, the nurse assumes the responsibility of assisting the client in meeting his or her health care needs. The nurse, in concert with other health care professionals, helps the client to understand what his or her needs really are, to know what possibilities are available for meeting these needs, to stand up to anyone who is threatening the client's autonomy or well-being, and to help the client help himself or herself. Thus the nurse makes it possible for a client to avail himself or herself of health care without having to lose the dignity and humanity concomitant with the exercise of autonomy. The client need not assume the role of the child. His or her status as a rational being is not threatened. Given the client's present condition (physical weakness, pain, anxiety, possibly confusion, and so on), the nurse is there to safeguard his or her status as an autonomous agent.

Nursing care, more than anything else, can contribute to diminishing the factors that (in many cases) inhibit the possibility of free, unfettered decision-making: the pain, the anxiety, the lack of knowledge of one's prognosis, one's alternatives, one's rights. If a client advocate instead of a parent surrogate, the nurse does not decide for the client. Rather, whenever possible, the nurse helps the client to decide. When that is not possible, the nurse takes those steps (a) which are likely to maximize the possibilities for the client's autonomous choice in the future or (b) which best express the client's wishes or aspirations (previously expressed by the client or inferred from past actions or information obtained from the client's family).

As mentioned, being a client advocate at times may entail standing up to other health professionals who are acting in ways that do not conform to the client's wishes or maximum autonomy. The nurse may also have to help the client so that she or he can insist on an alternative form of treatment or discontinuation of treatment or whatever. Indeed, it is also likely that the presence of nurses as effective client advocates would soon modify the behavior of any other health professionals who are inclined to act out of disregard for their client's autonomy. Quite likely they too would want to avoid unpleasant controversy and would take that into account in making their initial judgment. So the large number of unpleasant confrontations that are often imagined if nurses were generally to act as effective client advocates are just not at all probable. The claim that the delivery of health care would be hampered by nurses acting as client advocates just cannot be substantiated.

The nurse is ideally situated to perform the function of client advocate. The nurse's caring functions—attending to basic and intimate physical needs—put him or her in constant, close contact with the client. Frequently no other health care professional has anywhere near the same opportunities to observe and interact with the client. The nurse's professional training and position make it more possible for her or him than for family members to strike a balance between sensitive involvement with the client and a dispassionate, detached relationship. The nurse's training and experience also provide her or him with indispensible knowledge about prospects for cure, alternative modes of treatment, anticipated side-effects of treatments, and so on.

The conception of the nurse developed above is the one assumed by the framers of the ANA *Code of Ethics*. The nurse's first or primary obligation is to the client. And the fundamental responsibility to the client is respect for his or her "human dignity" and "uniqueness." This corresponds with the view developed in Chapter 1, in which we argued that the respect for persons principle has primacy. The nurse *qua* nurse, on this view, also takes this principle to be basic. It is the standard by which all of her or his activities are judged.

One of the most-controversial and divisive issues within the nursing profession in recent years has been that of educational requirements for the nurse [Fields, 1980a,b]. If the view of client advocate outlined here is to become the dominant model for nursing care, it is obvious that the nurse must be well educated. Nursing education must include teaching of basic nursing skills and technique but also nursing specialties, use of sophisticated equipment, and a broad understanding of the humanities, ethics, communication skills, and psychology. Precisely how the required education can best be accomplished is one of the main items on the agenda of nursing educators. What complicates the debate is the vested interests of the various types of degree programs, as well as the understandable concern of many graduates of diploma and associate degree programs when proposals are made to require nurses to have the baccalaureate degree to qualify as a "professional" nurse. If one considers oneself a professional and has for many years, to be placed in the bottom tier of a two-tier system and to be called a technical nurse is tantamount to a demotion. Also, such a person may be far better trained—through on-the-job experience and self-education—than those with baccalaureate degrees who are beginning their nursing careers. Accommodation, sensitivity, and creativity in dealing with these cases and in setting interim standards are not only necessary from the point of view of prudence (achieving the necessary good-will and votes to obtain the goal) but also from the point of view of morality (treating diploma and associate degree nurses fairly and with respect). Yet this does not in anyway reduce the need for a rigorous and broad educational requirement.

Beside the fact that a liberal arts education combined with rigorous nursing courses and experience is likely to be the most-efficient and effective way to gain the knowledge required to function effectively as a client advocate, another reason for establishing these (as is being done) as requirements for future entrants into the profession is that it is probably the only way nursing can achieve a standing of equality with other professions. That one can enter the profession of nursing without having completed a quality liberal arts education is a factor that sets nursing apart from most other professional groups. This is a dubious mark of distinction—and one that acts as a millstone around the neck of the profession.

If nurses are to be client advocates, their training also must instill a clear and affirmative self-concept. That is, they must understand and acknowledge their *own* moral rights. On the mother surrogate model and especially the handmaiden of the physician model, it is quite possible (even if not desirable) for the nurse to accept a subservient, even servile, role, to view herself or himself as standing lower than others, and to take a deferential attitude toward others due to ignorance or lack of understanding of one's own moral rights. But if one combines such an attitude with the client advocate model, it becomes a fatal flaw.

The fundamental moral principle upon which the client advocate model rests is the Kantian principle of respect for persons. This principle requires that each and every person be seen as having equal basic human rights. Each and everyone includes oneself. If a person is either blind to, or careless about, his or her fundamental rights, we would not be sanguine about having such a person as our advocate. We would want someone whose behavior reveals a deep understanding and profound respect for the demands of morality.

Acknowledging fully one's own rights as a person and developing a concept of oneself as a moral agent may be the first steps to recognizing and honoring the rights of others. The training of a nurse should include moral education to encourage and promote such personal growth. One of the positive features of feminism has been that it has acted as a catalyst for many women and nurses, helping them to see the moral defects of servility [Hill, 1973]. A person with a developed moral sense satisfies one of the essential criteria for being an effective advocate for a sick person. Combine this with knowledge of the various basic technical skills, nurse specialties, related disciplines, and so on, and we have a nurse who meets all the conditions for effective client advocacy.

In the remaining chapters of this book, we shall derive the nurse's role-related duties from the client advocate model. Not only is the client advocate model one that is gaining wide acceptance, we have seen that it is favored by the ANA *Code of Ethics*. Our discussion has made clear that the client advocate model is also firmly based on the fundamental moral principle of respect for persons derived in Chapter 1. Therefore, it is a very attractive model from the moral point of view. Nursing based on this model is a high calling, an exciting and fulfilling—but also demanding—way of life.

We have discussed the need for rigorous and broad training to meet the demands of contemporary nursing. We have considered various reasons why today's nurse needs a more thorough education than did the nurse of yesterday. But I wish to conclude this chapter with a caveat. Preoccupation with credentials and education can result in a failure to recognize or to be able to admit the limitations of one's knowledge—both one's own and that of the profession in general. The more diverse and specialized nursing becomes, the more difficult it is for a single individual to know all she or he may feel should be known. Socrates (470–399 BC), the patron saint of philosophy, was once told that he was the wisest of men. He found this hard to believe; all around were people who claimed to know many things of which Socrates knew he was ignorant. Yet it was true that Socrates was the wisest, for he (in contrast to the others) knew that he did not know many things. Knowing you do not know something puts you in the position to find out about it, to ask others about it. If you mistakenly think you know or are unwilling to admit ignorance, you are not in a position to learn.

Especially at this time when nursing is struggling to upgrade its image and its role, there will be a strong tendency for nurse educators and nurses on duty to want always to appear knowledgable, informed, and fully in control (a trait carefully nurtured by many physicians, and one for which they are increasingly sharply criticized). In such cases Socrates' example can provide guidance.

3

The Nurse-Doctor Relationship

The subordination of nursing to doctoring mirrors society's expectations that women will defer to men, nurses to doctors. This is true even though nurses and doctors have independent as well as overlapping functions in patient care. Doctors and patients expect nurses to act as subordinates of the doctor; most nurses have been socialized to do so [Steinfels, 1977, p. 20].

Thus wrote Margaret Steinfels in a report on a 1977 conference on teaching ethics in a nursing context. This is an accurate description of the situation in 1977 and perhaps now. But for reasons cited in the previous chapter, we must hope that the description would be less true of nursing today than it was in 1977 and that it will be less true of the future than it is of the present. The role of nurse as client advocate is not compatible with subservience and dependency.

The traditional relationship of the nurse to the doctor, more than any other aspect of nursing, has determined the parameters of nursing practice. Generally, nurse licensure has accepted the favored power position of the physician and has rather narrowly and rigidly defined the role of the nurse to conform to it [V. L. Bullough, 1975, p. 30]. In practice the nurse's authority, expertise, and activity often far exceed the defined role. The result has been well described by Dr. Leonard Stein in a widely discussed 1967 article entitled "The Doctor-Nurse Game."

One rarely hears a nurse say, "Doctor, I would recommend that you order a retention enema for Mrs. Brown." A physician, upon hearing a recommendation of that nature, would gape in amazement at the effrontery of the nurse.

The nurse, upon hearing the statement, would look over her shoulder to see who said it, hardly believing the words actually came from her own mouth. Nevertheless, if one observes closely, nurses make recommendations of more import every hour and physicians willingly and respectfully consider them. If the nurse is to make a suggestion without appearing insolent and the doctor is to seriously consider that suggestion, their interaction must not violate the rules of the game. . . . The object of the game is as follows: the nurse is to be bold, have initiative, and be responsible for making significant recommendations, while at the same time she must appear passive. This must be done in such a manner so as to make her recommendations appear to be initiated by the physician [Stein, 1967, p. 699].

Many nurses and doctors play this game very effectively. Often they have learned their parts before entering practice, since the doctor-nurse game is a version of the male-female game played in societies such as ours which reinforce gender stereotypes.

The more we all are free to reject these stereotypes (e.g., that males are to be assertive and females to be passive), the less likely it is that there will be willing, experienced, and capable players of the game. But even if the game were not threatened by the changes in our society, including the changing attitudes concerning the proper role of women, we would have strong moral and pragmatic reasons for urging that the conditions which make it necessary to play the game be changed.

Few relationships require more trust and understanding than the nurse-physician relationship. Only when they work in concert can the clients' needs adequately be met. To leave communication to a system of indirect discourse requiring complex deciphering of subtle (and perhaps nonverbal) messages is inefficient and risky.

The cardinal rule of the game is that open disagreement between the players must be avoided at all costs. Thus, the nurse must communicate her recommendations without appearing to be making a recommendation statement. The physician, in requesting a recommendation from a nurse, must do so without appearing to be asking for it. . . . The greater the significance of the recommendation, the more subtly the game must be played [Stein, 1967, p. 699].

Were it not for the posturing, an open discussion of the possible alternative courses of treatment and their effects on the particular client would be possible. Not only would there then be less chance of misunderstanding and resultant poor client care; it is possible that together they could come up with a treatment plan far superior to what either was considering on his or her own. This seems likely especially because each comes to the situation with a different perspective and frame of reference.

Nurses and physicians have rather different formal training. Physicians are trained in the diagnosis and treatment of disease, whereas nurses are trained to be knowledgeable about the treatment of illnesses and the complications of side effects of various treatment modalities. Nurses are more inclined to consider the general well-being of the client, whereas physicians, with their rigorous training in the diagnosis and treatment of disease, focus on the disease process itself. Because of their 24 hour care as opposed to the doctor's brief, once-a-day visits, the nurse is likely to know more about the client as a person. The nurse's emphasis is on care of the person, while generally the physician's is (perhaps quite correctly) on cure of the disease. Treatment plans would undoubtedly benefit from combining these different perspectives into a coherent whole. Collaboration based on mutual respect for the professional contributions of the other is clearly the relationship that a rational client would want of doctors and nurses.

Of course, there are situations (as, for example, in certain types of emergencies or during surgery) not conducive to collaboration that require deliberation or an exchange of ideas. It is crucial in these situations that a clear line of authority be well established. Obviously, it would be foolish and naive to think that during the procedure itself one could question the line of command that has been established for efficiency of operation. In these situations time is of the essence. Noone would push the concept of collaboration to this extreme. Any deliberation must have taken place prior to the procedure or it must wait until later. The converse has occurred, however; these exceptional cases have been taken as the model of the physician-nurse relationship for all other non-emergency, routine, everyday cases. Since a clear line of command is useful in the few cases, it has been promoted as the pattern best utilized in all. What is needed is a recognition that one pattern is not appropriate for all types of situations. A team approach with consultation and deliberation is better in a wide range of cases, and a clear line of command is superior with regard to special procedures and situations in which time is of the essence.

A hierarchial structure (vividly protrayed by Stein in "The Doctor-Nurse Game") made rigid and non-communicative by defensive worries about status is unquestionably inferior to an arrangement which makes provision for candid interaction and exchange among professionals with diverse training and expertise. This kind of interaction need not lead to chaos or uncertainty as to areas of responsibility. Open discussion in a context of mutual respect is compatible with a hierarchial arrangement, which vests final authority and ultimate responsibility in one of its members (e.g., the physician in charge).

Although not at all a commonplace, some institutions have encouraged nurses and doctors to develop relationships based on mutual respect and candid exchange of views. The model of the nurse-physician relationship that has evolved has been labeled the *joint practice concept*. The nurses, doctors, and institutions pioneering with this concept are in a position to make a very significant contribution not only to upgrading the nursing profession, but also to improved client care. More than ever before, the health care system is in danger of falling under the tyranny of high technology and of losing the human aspects of client care. The more dominant the physicians' role, the greater the likelihood of falling into this trap. A more-central role for nursing is essential for maintaining the proper balance and perspective.

The joint practice approach is based on dialogue, the open exchange of ideas, and candid evaluation of recommendations leading to a course of action. One engages in dialogue with those one respects as persons. The joint practice approach not only is an effective approach, as we have seen, it is also one that has much to commend it from the moral point of view. A relationship of mutual trust and respect, one which can openly recognize the contribution of the other, is not possible for players of the nurse-doctor game. But such respect and forthrightness—requirements of the moral point of view—are possible with the joint practice approach.

What lies at the base of the physician's failure to consult the nurse is either a disregard for the personhood of the client or a lack of respect for the competence of nurses or, perhaps, both. Even if the doctor's appropriate focus is narrow, he or she ought to recognize that the disease under treatment resides in a person. The person must be attended to, and in this, the nurse can be the most important ally. If the physician fails to take account of the nurse's contribution (which, as we have seen, is one that concerns itself with the individual and his or her autonomy), he or she (perhaps inadvertently) fails to respect the client as a person. On the other hand, if the physician does treat his or her client as a person while ignoring the contribution the nurse can make, the physician will be attempting to do both the doctor's and the nurse's functions. There may be (unusual) cases in which the nurse is so incompetent that the doctor must step in for the benefit of the client and either legislate nursing regimen to be carried out by passive aids or go far beyond the usual routine of brief daily visits. But certainly such cases (which, of course, are not the norm) are not the basis on which policies should be formulated. Because physicians generally recognize the valuable contribution nurses can and do make to the welfare of their clients, want the best for the clients, yet have been socialized to see nurses as their inferiors (functionaries to whom they must appear superior), the doctor-nurse game is played. The problem lies in the physicians' perception of the nurse.

The doctor-nurse game can be criticized, as we have above, for its inefficiency and the unnecessary risk it generates to clients when the indirect communication of the game fails. But now we can see as well that the game must be criticized because it fails to treat the nurse in a morally acceptable manner. It is demeaning to the nurse: it requires the nurse to assume a status and character below that which is really hers (or his). Contrary to fact, the nurse must appear not to be the independent professional for which her or his training and experience prepared her or him.

Obviously, all things being equal, we ought not and would not allow ourselves to be put in a demeaning position. Even more emphatically, we can say that one ought never to treat oneself or another in a demeaning manner. This follows directly from our fundamental Kantian principle of respect for persons. Were our purpose that of finding fault, the physicians who treat nurses in the way described would undoubtedly come in for the harshest criticism. Yet we would be remiss (in a book on moral problems in nursing) not to point out that—if it is possible to do so—nurses also have an obligation to try to change the situation. This, of course, is not something one can do by oneself; it requires collective action. In later chapters on collective responsibility (Chapters 6 and 7) we shall consider the question of nurses' collective obligation to see to it that individual nurses who find themselves in demeaning relationships will be able to count on their colleagues, their professional organizations, and their supervisors for support.

At present, rigorous support of a nurse in the difficult situation is unlikely. But even without full support from colleagues, professional organizations, and nurse supervisors, some change for the better is occurring. Slowly nurses are moving to a position or status closer to that befitting their calling and abilities. Yet the hospital nurse in particular is likely still to be a great distance from the goal of an *independent* professional. For many hospital nurses the reality of the situation is that they are expected to follow physicians' orders—orders for treatment plans to which they have had little or no opportunity to contribute.

Many scholars concerned with nursing ethics see the issue surrounding the obligation to follow orders as the central and special problem of nursing ethics. Beauchamp and Childress say, for example: "What is special about nursing from a moral point of view is the question of authority and power on the health care team" (Beauchamp & Childress, 1979, p. ix). For at least the traditional hospital nurse, moral concerns about following physicians' orders are of greatest urgency. Nonetheless, concern about how to relate to authority need not be the central problem for nursing per se. As we have seen, nursing can be and is practiced in different settings and with different models. In these other circumstances the question of authority and the problems of the nurse-physician relationship are not central.

Setting aside the question of the desirability of (and, indeed, necessity of) change in the nurse's role and status and also setting aside the fact that the situation is different in many nonhospital settings, let us consider the question of the proper response by hospital nurses to physicians' orders. As a matter of fact, nurses, physicians, and clients seem to presume that physicians' orders are to be followed by nurses. If a physician gives an order and—for whatever reason—the nurse does not follow it, she or he would feel that the burden is on her or him to demonstrate why it is not being followed. The physician is seen as having authority over the nurse when it comes to client care. The nurse is seen as obligated to carry out the orders of the physician. Yet we can at least imagine situations in which most would agree that a nurse ought not to follow a physician's orders; for example, when the order is obviously an error that could cause great harm or death to the client.

As we consider the cluster of problems that arise from the fact that physicians do give orders to hospital nurses, we shall discover that the usual way of looking at the nurse's supposed obligation to obey the physician is unacceptable. Nevertheless, let us begin by accepting (for purposes of discussion) the commonly held view that the nurse has a clearly established and stringent obligation to obey the physician's order. With this assumption in place we want to consider (A) When, if ever, is a nurse justified in refusing to follow a physician's order?

If we assume that the nurse has an obligation to obey the physician, the most likely type of situation which would call for an exception to the rule that physicians' orders must be obeyed by nurses would be when some other, more-stringent moral duty conflicts with the duty to obey.

In the example just cited, assuming that a nurse has a duty to protect a client from grave harm, an erroneous physician's order which, if followed, would result in great harm would be the sort of order the nurse would be justified in not obeying. In extreme cases such as this, the duty to the client, it could be argued, takes priority over the duty to obey the physician.

If an argument of this sort is to be used to show that, in some cases, disobeying a physician's order is justifiable, a better way to consider the question of the nurse's proper response to the physician's orders would be to ask (B) Are there situations in which the nurse is *obligated* to question physicians' orders? The proper formulation of the question is not when may a nurse disobey a physician's orders but when must she or he do so.

If we approach the question of the correct response to physicians' orders considering the nurse as an extension of the physician, we will be inclined to ask it in form A. If we approach the issue with the concept of nurse as client advocate, we will be inclined to ask it in form B.

Question B leads to an even more basic question: (C) What is the basis of the doctor's authority and the presumption that her or his orders should be followed? Asking this question will make clear that the common presumption that, because of the doctor-nurse relationship, nurses have a general duty to follow physicians' orders is unacceptable.

Let us turn to a careful consideration of B and C, beginning with B. When should a nurse refuse to follow a physician's order? There are three logically possible answers: never, sometimes, always. We can readily see that the only plausible answer of the three is sometimes. Suppose we were to say that a nurse should always refuse to follow a physician's orders. That would require a very different institution from the hospital as it exists today in which the physician has the primary responsibility for the care to be given to the client. (Such a change may be desirable, but that is beside the point for the present discussion. Our concern in this section is with the situation as it is and the morally appropriate behavior for nurses who must face the situation as it is.) In many cases the only way the nurse can act for the best interest of the client is to cooperate in the treatment plan ordered by the physician. The nurse's own commitment to being a client advocate provides the foundation for carrying out all those physician's orders that are compatible with the client's desires and needs. Because of our confidence that most of the time most doctors will know what is best for their clients and will want the best for them, we can make a presumption that doctors' orders should be followed by nurses.

The basis for this presumption, it should be noted, is not the status or position of the physician relative to the nurse. The source of the presumption is the mutual concern for the welfare of the client and the inductive generalization that following the physician's orders usually is best for the client. If following physicians' orders were not usually beneficial, the presumption that physicians' orders should be followed would be inappropriate. Fortunately, such a dismal appraisal of current medical practice need not be made. Unless there are clear indications to the contrary, the odds are that following the physicians' orders will also be the alternative that is best for one's clients.

Considerations of physician competence and dedication may lead one to the other extreme, namely, that the nurse ought always to follow a physician's order. All we need do, however, is reflect on several actual cases in which physicians' orders clearly were not in the clients' best interest, and we shall see that the only reasonable position to take is that sometimes the nurse should refuse to follow a physician's order. With this established, we shall turn to the difficult task of determining what distinguishes cases in which the nurse is acting properly in following the physician's orders from those in which she or he is not.

First, so that we can agree that the position that a nurse must always follow a doctor's orders is untenable, consider the following case—a case in which it is clear that the nurse ought to refuse to follow the doctor's orders.

I was caring for a patient who was in serious distress from an asthma condition. It was obvious he needed medical attention. I called his doctor and she gave no medical orders over the phone but instead came immediately to the hospital. When the doctor arrived she was obviously intoxicated. She left several orders for the patient. Some of the orders appeared to me and the other nurses as appropriate and some were definitely inappropriate and would possibly be harmful to the patient if given as ordered.

The patient's care was uppermost in my mind, but I also knew that the legal responsibility to order specific medications was the doctor's. In this case the patient's doctor was obviously in no condition to review the orders with me and hear my opinion as to the reasons they were inappropriate. For the patient's safety, my knowledge of pharmacology made me certain I should not give them. The other nurses on the unit agreed with me.

I consulted with other doctors who were present and knew of the dilemma. They had observed the condition of the doctor and also agreed that the orders were inappropriate. They refused, however, to take or even suggest any steps to resolve the problem.

Finally, the nurses definitely decided we should refuse to follow the doctor's orders. The nurses took turns staying constantly with the patient. We used whatever nursing measures we could to ease his condition. The other nurses spent a long time telephoning until finally the chief of the medical staff was contacted. When he arrived he made certain the appropriate medical care was ordered. The patient soon had relief [Tate, 1977, pp. 64–65].

Here we have a case of a mistaken and dangerous order by a physician. Obviously, following the order would not be compatible with the nurse's role as a client advocate. It may not even be compatible with being a handmaiden of the physician, since, in this case, the best way to help the physician is to refuse to follow the erroneous order.

The March 1979 issue of *RN* reported the results of a survey conducted among nurses to determine when they would take action if they observed physician mistakes. Ninety-six percent would take action if the error were life-threatening; 93 percent, if it were one that could lead to permanent injury; 54 percent, if the error precluded a better alternative therapy; 32 percent, if the chosen therapy were unnecessary; 28 percent, if the tests were unnecessary; 28 percent, if the error precluded cheaper alternative therapy; and 24 percent, if the error resulted in unnecessary hospitalization. This survey shows that, especially with mistakes having serious consequences, nurses believe that challenging the physician is not only what they ought to do but sometimes they would do. If all the respondents also saw themselves as client advocates, the percentage of nurses taking action in the cases of error with less serious consequences would have been high as well.

In many cases it is unpleasant and even risky for a nurse to challenge a physician or question her or his judgment. The understandable desire to avoid trouble for oneself may contribute to the hesitancy to question a physician's order. The physician may respond very angrily and complain that the nurse does not know her or his place. Or, if the nurse must go beyond the doctor and take the case to the nurse supervisor, other physicians, a departmental chairman, or a policy or ethics board, she or he may not only be unsuccessful but may suffer reprisals from those whose judgment was challenged. At a minimum the nurse will be labeled a troublemaker.

The following case illustrates all too vividly the kind of response many nurses receive if they try to act conscientiously when confronted with physician error or negligence.

As a new staff nurse, I was caring for a seriously ill patient who had a cardiac monitor attached. I was the only first level nurse on the unit when I noticed a change in the wave pattern on the monitor. My expertise was not adequate to categorize the specific change and there was no one there on the unit to help me. I called the supervisor who said she was too busy to come to the unit but that I should call the resident physician. I asked the telephone operator to page him and I returned to the patient.

There was no apparent change in the vital signs but the patient's restlessness became quite obvious and concerned me greatly. Although the resident had not answered his page, I finally located him in the emergency room. All I could tell him was the wave was different and I thought he should come and check the patient as I was not experienced enough to interpret the change. In about thirty minutes, the vital signs began to change drastically and I placed an emergency call to the resident to come immediately. He still had not arrived when I had to place a general emergency call because of the need for cardiac resuscitation. By the time he arrived his only duty was to pronounce the death of the patient.

I was off for the next two nights and when I returned I talked with the supervisor about reporting the lack of response from the resident. I felt that an investigation would establish whether he was negligent in his care or if the staffing was inadequate to cope with emergencies. She told me to forget the incident, an investigation would cause me a lot of unnecessary discomfort and be time-consuming. Without her support I did not press the issue [Tate, 1977, pp. 60–61].

We would not be surprised were we to learn that the next time this new staff nurse was faced with a similar problem she did not even consider reporting it.

Yet she may be "damned if she does" report such cases but also be "damned if she does not." There is no safe haven or clear escape route. The failure to take action to counteract a physician's error or negligence can lead to legal trouble and consequences just as unpleasant for the nurse as those resulting from taking action.

The nurse can be held legally accountable for failing to act to safeguard the client in the event of obvious physician error, whether it be an error of omission or commission. A nurse negligence case in West Virginia in 1977 is a clear example of nurses being held legally liable because they did not act vigorously enough in bringing to the attention of the proper authorities the results of physician mismanagement. A young man had broken his arm in a fall. A cast had been put on and he was admitted to the hospital. Several days later, the nurses discovered that his arm was swollen, black, and exuding a foul-smelling drainage. His temperature was high and at times he was delirious. He could not hold down oral antibiotics. The nurse in charge called the doctor explaining what was happening. Inexplicably, the doctor took no action. No other steps were taken to modify the treatment the young man was receiving. Finally, when such action was taken, it was too late. These efforts failed. His arm had to be amputated. When this case appeared before the State Supreme Court, it ruled that the nurses were negligent. They should have gone beyond the attending physician and reported the case to the physician's departmental chairman.

Of the three possible responses to the dilemma of when a nurse should refuse to follow a doctor's orders, we have seen that always and never are obviously unacceptable. We must turn to the only answer remaining. If nurses are sometimes morally required to refuse to follow physician's orders, we must determine as precisely as we can what distinguishes cases in which orders should be followed from those in which they should not. We have seen that there can be no question that the nurse ought not to follow orders that are both mistaken and obviously not in the client's best interest. But we must move beyond the clear-cut cases to the more common, subtle, and puzzling ones.

Consider the following case:

A frail patient recovering from recent surgery has been receiving intra-muscular antibiotic injections four times a day. The injection sites are very tender, and though the patient now is able to eat without problems, the intern refuses to change the order to an oral route of administration of the antibiotic because the absorption of the medication would be slightly diminished. The nurse must decide whether to follow the order as it stands or continue through channels to try to have the order changed [Mappes, 1981, p. 97].

This is not a case of obvious unsound medical practice. From the nurse's perspective however—one that is concerned with the general well-being of the client and not just the treatment of the condition—the alternative treatment plan (administering the antibiotic orally) can be seen to be preferable. Is this an order that should be questioned? If the role of the nurse is that of client advocate, then the answer must be affirmative. Having determined which alternative is best for the client, the nurse must raise questions about any course of treatment that deviates from it to the detriment of the client.

Suppose it were the case that administering the antibiotic orally would result in a modest but significant decrease in the amount of antibiotic absorbed. Then it would not be clear that the oral route is preferable to the intra-muscular injections. Although the nurse may still feel it would be better to stop the injections and administer the antibiotic orally, if the physician considered the two alternatives and favored continuing the injections, the nurse would be obliged to proceed accordingly.

The difference in these two cases is the degree of certainty that the nurse has about the relative superiority of the alternative she or he favors over that of the alternative ordered by the doctor. If a presumption in favor of following physicians' orders can be made because generally doing so is in the best interests of the client, then the burden of proof is on the nurse who questions the order or refuses to follow it. The nurse must have a clear basis for not following the physician's orders. The nurse's best defense is one that demonstrates that an alternative is a more adequate way of helping the client.

We have seen that the morally appropriate response of a nurse to an order which results from physician error and which jeopardizes the client's welfare is to refuse to follow the order. The nurse, as client advocate, is committed as well to refusing to follow orders that fail to respect the client as a person and that undermine the client's right to self-determination. Consider the following case, drawn (as was the previous one) from Professor Mappes's essay "Ethical Dilemmas for Nurses: Physicians' Orders versus Patient's Rights":

A patient in the cardiac unit who was admitted with a massive myocardial infarction begins to show signs of increased cardiac failure. The patient and the family have clearly expressed their desire to the medical and nursing staff to refrain from "heroics" should complications arise. The patient stops breathing and the intern begins to intubate the patient, requests the nurse's assistance, and orders a respirator. Should the nurse follow orders or attempt to convince the intern to reconsider, calling the resident-on-call should the intern refuse? [Mappes, 1981, p. 99].

As Professor Mappes says in commenting on this and similar examples, the correct response is to refuse to follow the order. The client's right to self-determination is being threatened. "One of the rights expressly outlined by the American Hospital Association is in danger of being abridged. . . . No formal training in medicine is necessary to arrive at the conclusion that the patient's right of self-determination is endangered" (Mappes, 1981, p. 99). Client advocates certainly are failing in their advocacy if they do not come to their clients' defense in cases such as this.

In the following case what the nurse ought to do is not nearly as evident. Suppose you are witness to the following conversation:

"I really don't understand you," Dr. Lowell said. "You definitely have cancer of the bladder. We may be able to remove it all surgically, but even if we can't, chemotherapy or radiation treatments have a good change of success."

"I want none of those," Patricia Jensen said. "I believe that a high-fiber diet and pure, filtered water are more likely to help me. I don't want to be cut or poisoned or burned."

"You're crazy," Dr. Lowell said. "That won't do anything."

"I intend to try it. Even if I'm wrong, it's my life."

"I won't let you," said Dr. Lowell. "Anybody who thinks the way you do about cancer is out of touch with reality. That's one of the marks of mental illness. And I intend to have you declared mentally incompetent to make decisions about your own welfare. I shall speak to the psychiatrists on our staff and ask the hospital lawyer to arrange for a sanity hearing" [Munson, 1979, p. 214].

Now suppose that Dr. Lowell leaves, clearly intent on doing what he said he would do. Patricia Jensen asks you if you would be willing to intervene on her behalf and challenge Dr. Lowell's actions. Should you?

One factor which complicates this case is that one can reasonably doubt that Ms. Jensen is acting in her best interests. Suppose that we conclude that she is not. Then action we take to promote her best interests will conflict with action we take to guarantee the exercise of her right to self-determination. Which of these conflicting duties takes priority? If, as client advocate, the duty to protect the client's right to self-determination takes priority over the duty to promote the client's best interest, the nurse must challenge the doctor's decision through appropriate channels (beginning by discussing the case with Dr. Lowell).

Cases such as this one in which what the client wants and what is in his or her best interest are not the same require us to clarify the notion of client advocacy. Is the client advocate primarily concerned to promote the client's best interests or to protect the client's right to choose? Obviously the client advocate would like to do both. But when both cannot be done, one is forced to make a choice. Without reflection I believe that most of us would be inclined to opt for doing what is in the client's best interest rather than what the client wants. Yet, if we are going to be consistent with the moral position outlined in Chapter 1 (in which it was argued that respect for a person's autonomy is the most-basic principle) and the view of the nurse as client advocate advanced in Chapter 2 (in which it was argued that the central feature of the nurse's role was safeguarding the client's status as an autonomous agent), we must maintain that the duty to protect the client's right to choose takes priority over that of promoting his or her best interests.

It is important at this stage of the discussion for the reader to reflect carefully and to consider whether this is a conclusion she or he can accept. It follows from the conclusions drawn in earlier chapters, which may have then seemed acceptable. Now, consistency requires that the conclusion be accepted or that some part of the discussion upon which it is based be rejected. For example, the view of the nurse as client advocate as developed here may be re-examined. Or the claim that respect for autonomy is basic may be challenged, and some other theory, for example, utilitarianism, may be put in its place. The arguments of these chapters have been advanced with the hope that the reader will be convinced that the conclusions drawn are the correct ones. Whether they are successful is a decision each reader must make.

If the reader is not fully persuaded, he or she will want to continue keeping in mind the points of difference and determining how these differences will affect conclusions in subsequent chapters. If the reader concurs with the discussion to this point, he or she will want to continue to follow the argument with a critical eye, for there may be other conclusions that will raise doubts.

In this spirit, let us return to the case of Ms. Jensen. The conclusion that must be drawn on the basis of our discussion is that the nurse is obliged to challenge Dr. Lowell on behalf of Ms. Jensen. Dr. Lowell's action is threatening Ms. Jensen's autonomy. He wishes to impose upon her his view of what is best for her. Dr. Lowell's response to Ms. Jensen's expression of her wishes is to assert his authority over her because of his conviction that he knows what is best for her while she does not. Even if we agree with Dr. Lowell that surgery is the best alternative from the point of view of probability of successful treatment of the bladder cancer, if we believe that the client's right to self-determination is paramount, we must respect her choice.

Were we to discover that Ms. Jensen is acting on inaccurate information, we certainly could point this out to her. One could even explain to her that her decision is one with which he or she cannot agree. Such behavior respects the autonomy of the other; it treats the other as a person. But in this context, to threaten to declare another mentally incompetent is to deny the moral status of the other. It is to attempt to justify treating the other as a nonperson, to ignore that person's independence.

Many cases of conflict between the nurse and physician involve a dispute over the appropriate limits of physician authority. The physician—motivated by a strong desire to bring the full arsenal of medical skill to bear on the case—may fail to take as a relevant consideration the fact that it is not what the client considers to be the preferred option. Or the physician may simply assume that, if a client chooses any course other than the one recommended, the one considered to be "medically indicated," the client is not acting rationally or even competently.

Of course, there are more complicated cases including those in which we cannot be sure the client is competent or we do not really know what the client wants (e.g., the client wants contradictory things: does not want surgery which she agrees is her only chance for a cure, and also wants very much to be cured and to do all that is necessary to bring this about). These complex cases raise the issue of when, if ever, it is appropriate to go against a person's present or immediate desires or to limit a person's freedom of choice in order to protect or advance that person's best long-range interests. This is the question of paternalism, which shall be discussed in Chapter 5. There we shall argue that, although paternalism is generally unacceptable because it fails to show respect for another's autonomy, there are special situations in which this is not the case and paternalism is justified.

What we have established in this chapter is that the nurse is obligated to raise questions about doctors' decisions which not only run contrary to a client's best interests but also those decisions which violate the client's right to self-determination. The duty to act in these ways arises from the commitment of the nurse to be a client advocate.

At this point in the discussion a very obvious objection can and should be raised. Given the current situation of relative powerlessness of nurses, in many situations the lone nurse challenging a physician's order will simply lose her or his job and nothing more will come of it. How can one require a nurse to do that? Two nurses quoted in the article in the March 1979 issue of *RN*, referred to earlier, recommend the following: Mackert says, "If you go to your supervisor and the director of nurses, and the whole agency is unresponsive, then you might consider employment elsewhere. No one person can change the system" (Stanley, 1979, p. 27). Hemelt says, "I hope that before taking on the whole hospital politically, you assess the potential for success. There is no point in putting your neck on the line without some possibility of getting results. Its important to plan strategy and for nurses to support one another in this. Some nurses think it's hypocrisy, but it's realistic" (Stanley, 1979, p. 27).

We must concede that only a very unusual individual could stand up to the massive health care system or even a local hospital hierarchy and make an impact. Yet it is not acceptable first to calculate the effects of acting morally before deciding whether or not to do what is moral. In those cases (some of which were discussed above) in which it is clear what morality requires, it would be wrong to fail to do it because of a negative assessment of "the potential for success." One does not act morally in order to produce favorable results. One acts morally because one is obligated to do so, hoping that his or her moral actions also will make a difference. Nor can it always be morally justifiable—as Mackert recommends by implication—to allow physicians to continue giving improper orders and winning confrontations with nurses by their deciding to move on to other employment settings whenever the going gets tough.

Another point made by Hemelt is very important and right on target, namely, the need for nurses to support one another. We have been considering the nurse-physician relationship from an *individualistic* perspective. One reason for this is that it is the individual who must make the difficult decisions we have been discussing. But the nurse as a professional is not merely an individual faced with difficult decisions. He or she is also a member of the profession, a collective. This wider perspective—which is seldom considered in a discussion of the nurse-physician relationship—does temper the conclusions we have reached in this chapter. As we shall see in Chapters 6 and 7 concerned with collective responsibility, removing some of the burden from the shoulders of the individual nurse involved in the difficult situation adds to the burden of all other nurses. They, too, as professionals bear responsibility. They must stand behind the nurse who finds himself or herself in the line of fire. If there is no professional support and there are no effective channels for registering concerns and challenging improper practices, the individual nurse will only rarely be able to make any notable difference. For most nurses most of the time, it will be extremely difficult if not impossible to act as an effective client advocate—something the nurse as a professional is pledged to do. Although (I shall argue) the individual nurse cannot be held responsible for this larger failure, the profession (i.e., all the members of the profession collectively) can be.

As we have seen, the physician's authority over the nurse is not absolute or unlimited. The nurse's duties to the physician are based on a more-basic duty, the fundamental duty of the nurse to the client. Hospital hierarchies are arranged so that for nurses to carry out their duties to their clients they must act in concert with physicians. As the health care system has evolved, physicians have been assigned final responsibility for the client. The nurse's obligation to follow the orders of physicians, then, arises from the fact that generally the client is best served by having physicians' orders carried out. This is so not only because physicians generally do order what is best for their clients, but also because it is often in the client's best interest that a coherent treatment plan be administered. Nevertheless, if a physician asks a nurse to do something that is detrimental to the client or that violates his or her autonomy, the nurse has no moral obligation to obey those orders; on the contrary, he or she has an obligation not to.

4

The Nurse-Client Relationship

In the chapter on the role of the nurse, we concluded that the concept of client advocate was an appealing one and would be used as the basis for subsequent discussion. We discussed in a general way what it means to be a client advocate. The implications of nurse advocacy were further discussed in regard to the physician-nurse relationship in the previous chapter. In this chapter, we shall consider specific types of clients and examine the role of the nurse in these relationships.

The Nurse and the Abortion Patient

Nearly all thoughtful people in recent years have felt compelled to try to come to terms with the abortion question in its moral, political (legal), and religious dimensions. The issue has polarized communities and swept politicians both into and out of power. State legislatures and the U. S. Congress continually propose new legislation concerning abortions. The courts make legal judgments. Organized "pro-life" groups push for a Constitutional amendment. Opposing "pro-choice" groups argue that a permissive abortion policy (including governmental funding for abortions for poor women) is a necessary condition for equal rights for women. Religious groups draft documents defending and opposing various positions. The Roman Catholic Church actively and vigorously opposes the current abortion laws and practice. Philosophers put forth careful arguments for a variety of positions running the gamut from the most restrictive to the most permissive.

Beginning in 1970, when Hawaii (followed shortly thereafter by New York) became the first state in the union to adopt "abortion on demand" as legal policy (i.,e., making abortion a personal choice to be decided between a woman and her physician), through January of 1973, when the U. S. Supreme Court legalized abortion nationwide, and on to the present, millions of women in the United States have sought and obtained abortions. For this to be possible, social workers, physicians, administrators, nurses, and many others have worked in concert to provide the desired services. Of all the professionals involved in abortion work, "the nursing personnel clearly bore the heaviest burden" (Kane et al., 1973, p. 410).

The extent of the nurses' role varies from center to center. In some a nurse plays the important "gatekeeping" role. That is, the nurse does the initial screening of women who have come to the hospital or clinic seeking abortions. Nurses are frequently assigned counseling duties to assist the woman in clarifying her own feelings and, in some cases, in confronting guilt or despair. Nurses are often assigned the task of providing information and guidance concerning contraception. Nurses assist physicians with the abortion procedure and care for the client after the procedure is completed.

If (as is presently the case) abortion services are going to be provided, it is reasonable that these duties be assigned to nurses. As Christa Keller and Pamela Copeland state in "Counseling the Abortion Patient is More than Talk," "The combination of medical knowledge, social awareness and feminine understanding allows the professional nurse to be the natural person to whom the abortion patient will relate" (Keller and Copeland, 1972, p. 106).

In order to carry out these duties with competence, it is essential that nurses (a) have technical knowledge about the abortion procedure which can be communicated to the client, (b) have knowledge of the possibilities and limits of various birth control methods and are comfortable discussing these with the client, (c) have an understanding of the complex moral and legal issues that arise in regard to abortion, and (d) have an awareness of their own emotional response to women seeking abortions and to involvement in the abortion procedure itself.

Of these necessary qualities, many nurses find that they have the greatest difficulty with the last. The following accounts of nurses' reactions to their involvement in the abortion procedure are representative.

The experience of participating in any abortion procedure goes directly against the medical emphasis on the preservation of life. On the gynecology hospital floor amnio abortions are viewed by the nurses as the most upsetting experiences which occur and a symbol of abandonment by the medical staff. The ward nurses' comments speak clearly to the point of being left to cope with an upset patient who delivers late at night. The house staff, although technically available, made clear their preference to be in the delivery room where "live births" occur. The nurses found the physical contact with the fetus particularly difficult; it reminded them of the "premies" just down the hall and made them uncomfortable about their own potential future pregnancies. Light staffing on the night shift made a totally voluntary system of participation difficult.

For the operating room nurses, there is a more evident freedom of choice about participation in the procedures and also more support from the physician who is present and who bears primary responsibility. The D and E [dilatation and extraction] procedure was described as distasteful and many nurses preferred noninvolvement. Nurses who did participate felt best when they had some time to get to know the patient prior to anesthesia. The discussion meetings generated a plan of active support for the patients both before and after the procedure as well as open acceptance of the right of individual choice about participation.

Amnio abortions often require protracted and intense nursing care with physician involvement only in emergencies. The floor nurse must deal with the expelled fetus; even nurses in favor of abortion find this a lonely and difficult task [Kaltreider, Goldsmith, and Margolis, 1979, p. 236-38].

The passage below from another study of nurses' emotional reactions to abortion also makes clear that nurses are the ones who have borne the brunt of the burden.

The hypertonic saline procedure was most traumatic for the nursing personnel, since they were generally the only ones present when the patient aborted. They resented being left with this responsibility, which could be very traumatic indeed. One nurse reported that she observed the aborted fetus moving. When asked what she did, she reported that "she stood and cried until the movement stopped" [Kane, et. al., 1973, p. 410].

Of all the people directly involved with abortion, nurses are the only ones to have been *compelled* to participate. Physicians, including obstetrical residents, have had the option of deciding whether to participate in abortion work. No abortion client (with a possible exception to be mentioned below) is required to have an abortion if she does not wish to have one. Nurses have not always been permitted such freedom, however, and their autonomy has not always been respected.

(There may now be an exception to the rule that clients not be compelled to have an abortion. It has been reported that women with fertility problems [e. g., blocked Fallopian tubes] seeking to become pregnant by means of the recently developed embryo transfer method are required to agree to have an abortion if the resultant fetus turns out to be defective or abnormal. Women opposed to abortion who see the embryo transfer method as the only way to have a child of their own [which may be their fondest hope] may feel they have no alternative but to give consent to an abortion. Other women, initially comfortable with idea of aborting a defective fetus, may find that when actually faced with the choice they do not believe it is the right thing to do. These possibilities raise complex moral issues which must be addressed—but we shall set them aside here and return to the issue of nurses being required to participate in the delivery of abortion services without their consent.)

A study of one situation at a major hospital in Honolulu in 1970 in which nurses were not given the right to refuse to be involved in abortion work is reported in the *American Journal of Psychiatry.* "Whether she was in the operating room or on the floor, the nurse had to cover whatever case came on her service" (Char and McDermott, 1972, p. 68). The clearly manifested adverse effects of this are described in the report that we shall look at later. As a result of bad experiences such as this, it is now generally recognized that to order nurses to assist in abortion if they have expressed moral objections or doubts is counter-productive. It just does not work well to run an abortion service with unwilling and demoralized help.

Circumstances often make it very difficult to have a "totally voluntary system of participation." Staffing needs are not alway predictable. The unit may unexpectedly be short-handed. Special problems including emergencies may arise. Nurses on one unit may be called to another. To refuse to help in circumstances such as these may be extremely difficult and may be interpreted as an affront to colleagues and supervisors.

Despite these very real pressures, however, the moral questions remain: Is it wrong for a nurse supervisor to order a nurse to participate in a procedure she knows the nurse believes is morally wrong? Does a nurse have a moral right or perhaps a moral duty to refuse to participate in actions she considers morally unacceptable?

In the previous chapter we argued that the nurse should refuse to follow orders that she or he found morally unacceptable (e.g., orders which put a client in danger or violated her or his autonomy). Does it follow that a nurse who finds abortion morally unacceptable should refuse to follow any orders to participate? Isn't this just another example of an order that the nurse (who finds abortion morally repugnant) has no obligation to follow?

One way to attempt to reject this conclusion would be to make a distinction between an action *being* immoral and someone *perceiving* an action to be immoral. Obviously a person's "perception" may be in error. Especially with the abortion question, which is notoriously difficult, we may want to draw this distinction. Then the argument would be that the nurse should refuse to follow those orders that are, in fact, immoral, but that those she or he merely thinks are immoral (but may not be) must be followed. The complexity of the issue and the wide divergence of views on the morality of abortion would be offered as support for the claim that, on this issue, we cannot really get beyond individual opinions to a point where we can know whether abortion is ever morally permissible or not. So, in the area of abortion, the nurse is not on the same solid ground in refusing to follow an order as she or he would be in refusing to follow an order that we could all agree is harmful to the client.

Although this argument makes an important point, namely, that the abortion issue is one that is far more difficult to think clearly about (because of its complexity) than whether we may allow a client to suffer an injury, it is not persuasive to someone who places fundamental importance on autonomy for all. The principle of respect for persons, for their autonomy, requires that the nurse too be free to exercise her or his moral judgment. If people are to be treated as autonomous, they must be seen as having the ability and the right to make their own moral judgments and to think for themselves. Suppose an obstetrics nurse working in OB-GYN facilities has concluded that abortion is wrong. But we say, "Too bad. We do not think you have thought it through very clearly. You must help us despite your scruples." Clearly we are failing to treat her as an autonomous being. We are imposing our will on her and ignoring her rationality. Only if we recognize that she has the right to refuse to participate are we acting consistently with the duty to respect her autonomy and rationality.

We can conclude that a nurse morally opposed to abortion is justified in refusing to be involved. A far more difficult case, however, is that of a nurse who is generally in favor of abortion but finds selective cases to be morally repugnant and wishes to abstain from participation in those. We shall return to this issue later.

The position that nurses with moral objections to abortion may conscientiously refuse to participate is seen by some as conflicting with current law, which gives women the right to an abortion. (We shall look at the specifics of the law later.) It is argued that the right to refuse to participate must be tempered by the duty to support the law. If women have a legal right to an abortion, then (since they cannot safely self-abort) someone else, namely, the health professional, has an obligation to perform the abortion. If this were not so, the argument continues, the right to an abortion is an empty one. It is a right that may be impossible to exercise, for there may be noone available to do it. In short, the claim that no health professional who finds abortion morally repugnant is obligated to perform them entails that women, especially in certain areas of the country, may have an empty right; no health professionals in the area may be willing to provide the service.

The possibility that a woman will be unable to exercise her (current) legal right to have an abortion is a consequence of asserting professional autonomy. To this extent, the argument just cited is correct. In opposition, I wish to maintain, however, that this is a conclusion we must accept. To do anything else would be to compromise the commitment to autonomy.

The argument can be challenged as well on rather different grounds. Maintaining that having the legal right to an abortion entails that someone else has a duty to provide the service is not the only way to construe the right. Instead we can construe it as merely entailing that no one else may interfere with a woman's exercising of her right. In short, I am suggesting that the right to an abortion can be seen as a negative rather than a positive right—i.e., as a right that forbids interference rather than as one that requires assistance. We often construe the legal right to free speech in this way. If I have a right to speak, you may not prevent me from speaking. Nonetheless, my having this right does not require that you or anyone else help me to speak (for example, buy me a loudspeaker, give me diction lessons, write my speeches, or carry them on television). As long as no one interferes, we are left to our own devices in attempting to exercise the right.

Although it is quite understandable that proponents of legal abortions would wish to construe the right to abortion as a positive right, we have seen that it is not the only way the right must be construed. If it is construed as a negative right, then there is no incompatibility between affirming that abortion is a legal right of women and that health professionals may conscientiously refuse to perform abortions. Even someone supporting the legal right to an abortion can then also strongly object to the practice of nonvoluntary participation in abortion work.

(In the recent controversy concerning governmental payments for abortion of poor women, the side supporting payments sees the right to an abortion as a positive right and the other side as a negative one. [Of course, some who oppose payments are simply opposed to all abortions and deny that women have a moral right to abortion at all.])

It is interesting to note that in the Honolulu case introduced earlier, when many of the nurses assigned to assist with abortions reacted adversely to what they saw, the chief of staff of the hospital brought in psychiatric consultants to help them cope with the problem of nurses "threatening to quit their jobs." The basic concern was *not* to help the nurses or to respect their autonomy but to keep the hospital running smoothly. The psychiatrists called in gave the following report:

The nurses' strong reactions were a surprise to even some of them since many of them, including some of the Catholic nurses, appreciated the problem of unwanted pregnancies and had approved of the new abortion law before it went into operation. But once the nurses became personally, intimately, and constantly involved with abortions, their intellectual and professional objective attitudes favoring legalized abortions were replaced by deeply personal emotional reactions so strong that many of them were even questioning the wisdom of the new law [Char and McDermott, 1972, p. 67].

The psychiatrists stated, in an article that appeared in the *American Journal of Psychiatry*, that they successfully dealt with the problem: "Abortion is now considered a routine matter" (Char and McDermott, 1972, p. 70). Among the means used to resolve the problem was helping the nurses "regain objectivity about abortions." After their work, they reported that the nurses "saw again that what is aborted is a protoplasmic mass and not a real, live, grown-up individual." According to them, many of the nurses had "overidentified with the aborted fetus."

A most disturbing experience to the nurses was to hold a well-formed aborted fetus with movement and with its eyes "still alive." (Twelve- to 24-week pregnancies were aborted by the injection of saline into the uterus, causing labor in 12 to 24 hours and the subsequent expulsion of the fetus.) A severe anxiety-provoking factor in this experience was the nurses' intense conflict about what to do with the fetus. In the past they were trained to try to save a premature infant, and physicians could be immediately summoned to help them with this task. Now, on their own, they were supposed to discard the fetus, and yet their old training still tried to tell them to summon help to save it.

Pregnancies of less than twelve weeks' duration were aborted by the dilation and curettage (D and C) method. Some of the nurses overreacted when they allegedly saw formed fetal parts such as hair and bits of limbs being sucked out or scraped out. The nurses who overidentified with the fetus projected into the protoplasmic masses real, live, grown-up individuals [Char and McDermott, 1972, p. 67].

The response described here and labeled overreaction by the psychiatrists is a very common one not only for nurses, but for many others who either assist in or observe abortions (Selzer, 1975). An operating nurse says the following:

It isn't so bad when the embryo has been taken away before the form is recognizable as a human being. But it's hard for me to get accustomed to the situation where gestation has proceeded, say, on into the third month. You know there is no chance for such an infant, if it can be called that, to survive. Yet there it is, a recognizable boy or girl, and you know that you have been part of the operation that caused its life to be terminated. I can't say that I feel I am an accessory to murder. I wouldn't go that far. But I say that it shakes me up—and I cannot help asking myself whether this is right, just for any trivial reason that a woman might cook up [Branson, 1972, p. 106].

If the question of the morality of abortion were as simple and clear as the Honolulu psychiatrists think it is, this common reaction could be labeled overreaction. But, as we shall see, it is far more complicated. To state that the description of the fetus as a "protoplasmic mass" is the objective view or description of it is to beg the question. The nurses' problem is that their experience is at varience with the description. The experience forces us to consider other possible descriptions such as a "fetus having human form" or a "potential person," or perhaps even a "person." On these other descriptions it is not obvious that the nurses' reactions are overreactions. They may be. But some argument (such as philosophers try to provide) is required to support the contention.

The problem of giving a correct description of the fetus is analogous to giving a correct description of Homo sapiens.

And what are we to say of man? Is he a speck of dust crawling helplessly on a small and unimportant planet, as the astronomers see it? Or is he, as the chemist might hold, a heap of chemicals put together in some cunning way? Or, finally, is man what he appears to Hamlet, noble in reason, infinite in faculty? Is man, perhaps, all of these at once? [Russell, 1959, p. 8].

To say that any one of these descriptions of man (human beings) is *the* "objective" one would be presumptuous and parochial in the same way that saying the biochemistry description of a fetus as a "protoplasmic mass" is. The fetus may be a protoplasmic mass, but it is presumptuous to say that that is all it is. Is it not also, for example, a potential person?

The psychiatrists' approach to the problem must also be criticized on another score. They make a distinction between the nurses' "intellectual and professional objective attitudes" and their "deeply personal emotional reactions" (see the quotation above). They state that the nurses allowed their emotional reaction to interfere with their intellectual attitude. Their treatment plan is to restore the intellectual attitude to a superior position and to discredit their emotions.

Can we be so sure in matters of morality that our ratiocination and rationalization are better guides than our feelings and sensitivities? The best moral thinking must take account of *both* . On the one hand, we must test our principles by our moral feelings or intuitions and, on the other hand, we must constantly subject our moral intuitions to the challenge of reasoned principles. Only when both point in the same direction can we be confident of our moral view.

What makes the abortion question so difficult is that the sensitive person is pulled in very different directions. We have discussed some nurses' responses to the abortion procedure and their identification with the fetus. The nurse who empathizes with her clients will also have strong emotional reactions and will identify with women seeking abortions—especially in the cases in which abortions can prevent untold suffering, e.g., those that provide the chance for a teenager to continue in high school, or allow a mother of several children who are totally financially dependent upon her to continue to work, or help a frightened girl recover from the trauma of rape, or prevent the birth of a baby who would be inflicted with Tay Sachs disease. These very different responses must be subjected to reasoned principles, and the principles must be able to account for these responses. Every thinking moral agent must engage in this philosophical activity; the best way to do so is through philosophical discussion.

Philosophical discussion of the morality of abortion in print has been focused on two basic questions: (a) What is the moral status of the fetus? (b) What rights does a pregnant woman have relative to the fetus? If the first question is answered by arguing that the fetus has the same moral standing as a person—that is, by claiming that the fetus is a person—then determining the rights of the pregnant woman relative to the fetus is required, just as in any other conflict of interest involving two persons. Often people hold that the only sufficient justification for killing another is self-defense. On this view, the only justification for abortion would be self-defense; for example, continued pregnancy is threatening the life or fundamental well-being of the mother (English, 1975).

Other philosophers have argued that the fetus does not have the moral status of a person because it lacks the requirements for personhood—e.g., self-awareness or self-consciousness (Tooley, 1972). If the fetus is not a person, then treatment of it is not necessarily subject to the same constraints that apply in our interaction with other persons.

In thinking about this issue it is of utmost importance that one be clear about the meanings of the terms used to describe the fetus. Often people argue, for example, that the fetus is obviously a human from the moment of conception (it is not a cow or a pig). Therefore, it is a person. The unstated principle is that all humans are persons. This may sound reasonable. But if it is an assumption of the argument, no argument has been advanced. This just is the issue under dispute. The question is whether the class of all humanoids coincides with the class of persons. Clearly, the criterion for being a person could be quite different from that for being a human. All that may be required to be a human is to be alive and born of human parents. But we may wonder whether that is the criterion for being a person. Certainly we can imagine nonhuman persons. Many religions consider angels and God as persons. So being of human parentage does not appear to be a requirement for personhood. Can we also imagine nonperson humans? For example, is an anencephalic (human) infant a person? ("Anencephalic" means without a brain. It is a condition of markedly defective development of the brain so that only a rudimentary brain stem and some traces of basal ganglia are present.) Must at least some qualities that we usually attribute to persons be present (e.g., consciousness, the capacity to feel pain, reasoning, self-motivated activity, the capacity to communicate, self-awareness [Warren, 1973])?

The notion of "person" which we have been using in this essay in arguing that the fundamental principle of morality is respect for persons as autonomous beings is that of a being able to act with self-consciousness. As Immanuel Kant stated, "The fact that man can have the idea 'I' raises him infinitely above all other beings living on earth. By this he is a *person* " (Kant, 1947, p. 9). A fetus, then, fails to meet the minimal conditions for personhood.

A consequence of taking this position is that the abortion issue is not construed as a conflict between two persons similar to any other life-endangering conflict. Instead, in abortion we are dealing with a unique being; a human that is not yet a person. What is the morally proper way to deal with such a being? And how are we to regard its "interests" relative to those of the woman carrying it?

Clearly it does *not* follow that anything is permissible. Even if the fetus is not a person, it is a *potential* person. That is, it "is a being, not yet a person, that will become an actual person in the normal course of its development" (Langerak, 1979, p. 25). If we respect and value persons we would also see that it is appropriate to value potential persons. Although a potential person may have a weaker claim to life (just as a potential president, a president-elect, has a weaker claim to power than does an actual president), surely its potentiality provides support for its claim to respect. As Alan Donagan states:

If respect is owed to beings because they are in a certain state, it is owed to whatever, by its very nature, develops into that state. To reject this principle would be arbitrary, if indeed it would be intelligible. What could be made of somebody who professed to rate the state of rational agency as of supreme value, but who regarded as expendable any rational creature whose powers were as yet undeveloped? [Donagan, 1977, p. 171]

Some special consideration for the fetus as a potential person must be given it in adjudicating conflicts of interest with its "mother." What is not settled by the fact that the fetus is a potential person is "the question of just how strong a claim to life should be attributed to the fetus" (Langerak, 1979, p. 26). Whatever their strength, these claims are countered by those of the "mother," an actual, autonomous person. As we have seen in earlier discussions, autonomy and self-determination are highly valued. These are often what are at issue when a woman seeks an abortion. When decisions have to be made concerning when, if ever, abortion is morally permissible or should be made legally permissible, these competing claims or interests must be weighed.

The United States Supreme Court tried to find a reasonable way to balance these interests and thereby establish firm ground for legal policy. The Supreme Court decisions of January 22, 1973 (*Roe v. Wade* and *Doe v. Bolton)* are the watershed in the legal aspects of the abortion controversy in the United States. In *Roe v. Wade* , the Court legalized abortion nationwide. The Court ruled that during the first three months of a pregnancy a decision to have an abortion must be left to the woman and her doctor. During the pregnancy's second trimester states may interfere in that decision only to protect the woman's health. In the third trimester the state may take steps to protect fetal life.

The Supreme Court based its judgment on the legal notion of privacy—the principle of autonomy, liberty, and noninterference. If the state is going to overrule the strong but qualified right to privacy, it must have a "compelling state interest" in so doing. The Court maintained that the state had "important and legitimate interests" in (a) preserving and protecting the health of the pregnant woman and (b) protecting the potentiality of human life. The state's legitimate interest in preserving and protecting the health of the pregnant woman becomes "compelling" only after the first trimester. Before that, the dangers are not great enough to warrant state interference. After the first trimester (twelve weeks), because the risks of abortion increase, states are permitted to set requirements (such as that a hospital is the only place an abortion may be performed) for safety's sake. The state's legitimate interest in protecting the potentiality of human life becomes "compelling" only after the second trimester or (which the Court designates as the same time) the point of *viability* —the point at which the fetus is "potentially able to live outside the mother's womb, albeit with artificial aid."

Two questions immediately arise for health professionals providing abortion services under these legal parameters: Which of the two criteria for the state's compelling interest in protecting fetal life— twenty-four weeks or viability—is basic? Why is viability a relevant consideration? Put another way, what is it about viability that makes it a nonarbitrary point at which to draw the line between permitting and prohibiting the termination of fetal life? Whether explicitly raised by those performing abortions or not, it is clear from the anxieties and concerns that have been expressed by thoughtful and sensitive nurses that these questions are basic. Puzzlement about these issues is the way the question of the morality of abortion continually arises for those involved in abortion work, challenging them to reconsider their moral stance.

Especially because of the fast pace of recent developments in neonatal care, the fact that the viability criterion is relative to time and place and dependent in large measure on changing technology and other external circumstances makes one uneasy. Acting in accordance with the viability criterion seems to have the implication that late-term abortions presently legally condoned by appeal to the 24-week criterion should no longer be performed. The problem is acute for nurses who work in both an abortion unit and in neonatal nurseries, in which heroic efforts to save ever younger and smaller prematurely born infants succeed. The difference of treatment of fetuses of identical age, size, and development seems arbitrary and capricious.

A more-fundamental problem with the viability principle is that by itself it does not seem to offer us a morally relevant difference. According to the viability principle as it is applied to abortions, the life of a nonviable fetus—that is, one which is dependent upon its "mother" for survival—may be taken. But the life of the viable fetus—one that is "potentially able to live outside the mother's womb, albeit with artificial aid"—may not be taken. Why this difference per se should warrant such radically different treatment is puzzling. Why does this difference give the one a "right to life" while the other is denied that right?

Whether the individual undergoing treatment is viable is a crucial question in clinical judgments concerning resuscitation of neonates and critically ill clients.

In treatment decisions, the physician is considering the use of expensive and possibly painful medical intervention to prolong the patient's life. The relevance and importance of viability is obvious: if the patient is not viable, the intervention is pointless and ought not to be carried out [Fost, Chudwin, and Wikler, 1980, p. 12].

With the nonviable fetus the issue is not that intervention is pointless. Nonviability is claimed to be grounds for permitting intervention that will result in its termination. But we are without an explanation as to why viability is a *morally* relevant criterion for treating viable and nonviable fetuses differently. What we need is some nonarbitrary criteria for drawing the line.

Professor Edward Langerak has suggested two basic criteria for moral and legal line-drawing: "important shifts in probabilities and dangerous social consequences" (Langerak, 1979, p. 27). The greater the probability of a fetus becoming an actual person, the stronger will be its claim to life. "The probability of an older fetus becoming an actual person is perhaps double the probability of a zygote becoming a person" (Langerak, 1979, p. 26). Hence, the strength of a defense for a late-term abortion must be considerably greater than that for a very early abortion. On the continuum of growth from conception to implantation to viability to birth, the probability of becoming a person (as we have seen "person" defined) increases, and so does the strength of the claim to life. Also, as we have seen, the more advanced the development of the fetus and the greater its odds of surviving on its own, the more brutalizing on the staff is performing the abortion and the more dangerous are the social consequences. Hence, viability seems to be the *outside* boundary for any morally permissible abortion, except for those rare cases of self-defense, narrowly construed. Because of these two factors (probability shifts and social consequences), the closer the fetus is to the point of viability, the greater the burden of justification. Also because of these factors, as medical advances move the point of viability to earlier times, the span within which abortions are permissible diminishes.

Under current law, a nurse who holds a moderate view of the morality of abortion (that is, who believes some cases of abortion are morally justifiable but others are not) is in the most difficult position if asked to assist in abortion work. The conservative nurse who is opposed to all or nearly all abortions (either because she sees the fetus as a person or believes that only rarely can the interests of the "mother" outweigh those of the fetus, the potential person) is in a strong position to refuse to work in the abortion unit. We have argued that that refusal must be respected. The liberal nurse who is convinced that all abortions requested by a pregnant woman prior to the point of fetal viability are permissible (because she believes that only rarely can the interests of the fetus outweigh the "mother's" right to self-determination) will have no moral difficulties in assisting with any (legal) abortions performed at the abortion center.

No conflict arises between the client seeking an abortion and either the conservative or liberal nurse. The client will not interact with the conservative at all. The liberal nurse will have no problem being supportive and being a client advocate. The moderate will find herself unable, in certain cases, to support the decision to have an abortion. For example, the moderate could not concur with a decision to have a mid-trimester abortion (say) for the sole reason that the fetus is a female (a fact determined by amniocentesis) and the couple desires a male heir or wants only two children, one of each sex, and already has a girl. A moderate would have deep concern about women who allow abortion to be their first or sole means of birth control, a practice that has produced the "abortion-repeater syndrome." According to a New York Times report: "Almost two of every five women having an abortion in New York City have had one before—or two, or four, or five, or, in one exceptional case, fourteen." A few years ago, of the 1,526 abortions performed at New York Hospital, 701 were repeats (*New York Times*, September 19, 1979).

Should the moderate follow the lead of the conservative and conscientiously refuse to participate in abortion work altogether? Or should she refuse to participate selectively? Blanket refusal to participate would cause no problem as long as others willingly participate. Surely this is a better alternative than "going along" with practices one finds morally repugnant. Drawbacks to this approach are that one no longer has any input into how the service is delivered and one is in a weaker position to effect change. Also, one may not want to give up one's job in the abortion unit because of the (perhaps relatively few) objectionable cases one might encounter. This, then, suggests the alternative of selective conscientious refusal.

In order to act in accordance with one's moral principles, it may be necessary to refuse to participate in a case that comes before one. But an abortion unit would not be well run were too many professionals to do this too often on a case-by-case basis. Especially if nurses acting as counselors were to do this with each case as it came along, it could have quite an adverse effect on clients. Selective conscientious refusal to participate could work if each nurse were to make clear ahead of time which *category* of cases she finds morally repugnant. If, in following this approach, a unit were to find that none of its staff approved of certain categories of abortions, they would be obliged to let it be known that they could not provide that service at their facility. They would not be obliged to offer the service.

The question of the morality of abortion is notoriously complex. It would take far more discussion than the space allotted here fully to come to terms with it. We have seen what the major positions and issues are, however. An outline of a defense for my own moderate position has been presented. Realizing that nurses' individual experiences and reflection lead to very different positions concerning the morality of abortion, guidelines for participation or nonparticipation in abortion work have been offered.

The Nurse and the Care of Defective Newborns

Nontreatment of defective newborns has occurred throughout history, but only recently has the medical profession openly acknowledged the scope and alleged desirability of the practice. In 1973, Doctors Raymond S. Duff and

A.G.M. Campbell documented 43 cases of withholding care from defective infants at the Yale-New Haven Hopsital, thereby breaking what they characterized as "public and professional silence on a major social taboo." Subsequently, similar cases across the country have received widespread public attention. Recently, the Senate Subcommittee on Health held hearings at which eminent physicians attempted to justify the practice. Pediatric textbooks discuss clinical indicators for withholding treatment, and physicians writing in medical journals have advocated nontreatment in certain situations. Thus, nontreatment of defective infants, now occurring in hospitals throughout the United States and England, is rapidly gaining status as "good medical practice" [Robertson, 1975, p. 213].

The greater sophistication of recent medical technology (e.g., contemporary resuscitation and life-saving devices) has made the question of the proper treatment of defective newborns a more complicated and difficult one than it was only a few decades ago. We are able to save (i.e., keep alive) more and more premature babies at increasingly early stages of pregnancy. In some cases the results are very gratifying. In many others, however, the results are tragic—infants survive with severe and painful defects and with virtually no chance of achieving even such minimal qualities of life as self-awareness. Surgical procedures developed in recent years can dramatically save defective infants who otherwise would not have survived beyond a few hours or days. In some cases the surgery is a godsend, but in others it is a nightmare.

Nurses' involvement in the decision-making concerning the treatment of defective newborns varies considerably. In some settings (to take one end of the spectrum) nurses are part of the team that—in conjunction with the parents—deliberates and decides what is to be done. In other settings (to take the other end of the spectrum) nurses are simply presented with a *fait accompli*: the doctors, perhaps the parents, or both, have decided not to treat, and the defective newborn is handed over to the nursing staff, whose job is to care for it in its final hours, days, or weeks.

We shall look at cases from both of these types of settings. After considering the various moral issues raised by the cases, I shall argue that nurses must work to avoid being put in the position of having to carry out decisions concerning treatment of defective newborns about which they have had no say.

If a nurse is relatively clear about the issues and, for the most part, concurs with the judgments made by physicians and other colleagues, it is possible—as in the following nurse's account—to serve with effectiveness and with a sense of satisfaction.

Spina-bifida is an operable condition. Depending on the degree of deformity an operation can be successful and lead to a life which is useful and happy or it can lead to something tragic—a child so grossly damaged and deformed that the quality of life is not acceptable by most standards of humanity. A life sentence of suffering has been passed not only on the child himself, but on parents and siblings as well. Today pediatricians are selective. Not all these babies are treated. It is an agonizing decision for them to make.

Parents are asked what they wish done but their knowledge is, of necessity, so limited that they can only do what the doctors seem to advise. Nurses are given the care of a baby who will eventually die, but how soon? One doctor with whom I worked felt that this should be as soon as possible. He said society has denied the child the possibility of meaningful life, and we should not prolong suffering—if, indeed, the child does suffer. He would request that we feed them on water only and give some sedation. Those I nursed were given care and love, and I made a point of doing as much of the care as I could myself. I always hoped parents would not wish to visit, but most did choose to see the baby. I did not encourage handling and I did not talk about feeding. Many of the parents wished their baby to be baptized; a minister or priest was called and we all attended. I gave priority to supporting the parents in their bereavement while the baby lived. I also felt it important to talk to all the younger nurses about the problem and the nursing care, giving them an opportunity to discuss and possibly object. None ever said much, and none objected, but I did not think that all nurses felt able to co-operate in such a course of action.

My own convictions allowed me to cooperate fully with the pediatrician. To me the greatest tragedies of medicine today occur when life is prolonged when it should be allowed to cease. Due to modern science it is possible, for example, to drain the fluid from the head of a hydrocephalic patient when it is obvious that the brain must already be grossly damaged and never likely to recover. This, to me, is an error. If a normal person is unsuccessfully resuscitated, and left handicapped it is unfortunate. However, if that happens we have done our best in good faith and should not reproach ourselves. In the case of a spina-bifida, I believe the matter is quite different [Tate, 1977, pp. 4–5].

The situation was quite different for nurses in the infamous Johns Hopkins case in 1972, described here by Anthony Shaw:

The lingering death of a newborn infant whose parents have denied consent for surgery can have a disastrous effect on hospital personnel, as illustrated . . . by the well publicized Johns Hopkins Hospital case, which raised a national storm of controversy. In this case, involving an infant with mongoloidism and duodenal atreasia, several of the infant's physicians violently disagreed with the parents' decision not to allow surgery. The baby's lingering death (15 days) severely demoralized the nursing and house staffs [Shaw, 1973, p. 886].

Despite the nearly uniformly negative criticism of the handling of this case, many similar cases continue to be handled in a similar fashion. As in this case, doctors frequently feel that the decision whether to treat a defective newborn should be left to the parents. Particularly if the parents do not wish to have the newborn treated, the physicians are hesitant to thwart the parents' decision through a court order (Freund, 1977). Without a court order, they must, of course, have parental consent in order to intervene. (In the Johns Hopkins case, the doctors were especially reluctant to challenge the parents' choice, because the mother was a nurse who had at one time worked with defective children. Presumably, if any parents would be in a position to have a clear understanding of the situation, these parents would.)

Surely one of the fundamental questions that must be addressed when considering the morally proper course of action with regard to defective newborns is: *Who* should decide? In earlier times, as a general rule physicians were far too prone to see themselves as the only ones qualified and authorized to make life and death decisions. The team concept (discussed in earlier chapters) modifies this autocratic approach by ensuring that the various health professionals involved in the case as well as the parents will have a chance to contribute to the decision. But perhaps, as is pointed out by the nurse quoted above who described her work with defective newborns, the team approach still leaves too much of the actual decision-making in the hands of the physician, given his or her position of influence and power. Recently, however, as is evidenced in the Johns Hopkins case, the pendulum has swung to the side of parental choice. Rather than being paternalistic, the health professionals carry out the wishes of the parents, despite their own reservations and uneasiness. Obviously, a middle course between these two extremes is preferable.

For those concerned with maximizing autonomy and counteracting the tradition of medical paternalism, letting parents decide may appear to be a much needed antidote. Of course, what complicates the issue is that the parents are not the client—the defective newborn is. But he or she is without voice or vote. Parental consent is proxy consent. An obvious answer to why a competent client should decide his or her own case is that it is his life and to deny him this choice would be to violate his autonomy. This answer, however, does not answer why the parents should be the ones to decide for the defective newborn. Since they are deciding *for another* , we must ask (1) whether they, of all the possibilities, are the best qualified to make this kind of decision, and (2) whether they are the most likely to have the best interests of the child at heart. If we cannot answer these in the affirmative but still wish to maintain that it is the parents who should decide, is it some special factor about the parents that makes them the proper ones to decide? (3) Do they "own" the child? (4) Or does the fact that they would most likely be the ones to have the burden of caring for it (which may be very costly emotionally, monetarily, socially, and so on) give them the right to decide? Or is the policy of parental decision-making vital for (5) maintaining the integrity and strength of the family as an institution or (6) maintaining the autonomy of parents?

To determine the nurse's proper role in the decision-making process, we must come to terms with these questions concerning the proper parental involvement. Depending on how we decide these issues, we will see the nurse's role as, for example, one of supporting the parents in whatever they decide, or very differently as one of protecting the interests of the defective newborn, whose care is most directly their responsibility.

Let us carefully consider what arguments can be given for and against vesting the final decision-making power in the hands of the parents. We shall take the reasons just cited for doing so (1–6) and consider whether they are persuasive.

1. Are the parents the best qualified to make the decision? As a general rule, we would have to say that they are not. They know little about birth defects, taking care of defective children, the possibilities for training such children, support services, and so on. Nor are they in the best position to make a decision of this magnitude after the traumatic experiences they have just gone through. (Think of the disappointment of the parents who were expecting a bouncy, healthy, cuddly baby.) Particular cases may be different, as the physicians felt was the case in the Johns Hopkins case cited above. Even in that case, however, there is some question whether the parents really knew the range of possible intelligence levels of children with Down's syndrome, what support services were available and many other relevant facts.)

2. Are the parents the most likely persons to have the best interests of the child uppermost in their thoughts? Surely in some cases there is no doubt that they do, yet, many factors could stand in the way of such altruism. Of all the parties involved, no others have so much at issue; treating a defective newborn could lead to their being forced to alter their life style, their hopes, and their dreams. Since it is likely to have an adverse effect on so many other areas of their lives (e.g., their careers, other children in the family, travel plans, hopes of buying a home) it may be especially difficult for them to focus on the best interests of the newborn. (There may be nothing wrong with their considering their own conflicting interests and even giving them greater weight than those of the newborn. Nevertheless, the fact that they are likely to do so challenges the parental altruism rationale for vesting the decision-making power in their hands.)

In an earlier age we were more inclined to accept (as a given) the notion of a natural link between parental interests and the child's best interests. David and Sheila Rothman in "The Conflict over Children's Rights" point out how the women's rights movement and more permissive policies and attitudes toward abortion have challenged the assumption of the identity of interest between mother and child.

Once women began proclaiming their independence from the role of mother . . . it became apparent to many observers that the identity of interest between mother and child was no longer operative. In this sense, the children's rights movement gathered added strength as an antidote to the women's rights movement. If women were determined to pursue their own interests, whatever they might be, then who would pursue the best interests of the child? The legalization of what was once the mother's cardinal sin could not help but symbolize just how far the post-1960 generation had moved from inherited doctrines. If one could now posit that a woman had rights over a fetus, how maintain the view that mother and child shared a harmony of interests? When the feminist movement so strongly advocated abortion and so many women were prepared to use the procedure, the nineteenth-century sense of a natural link between woman's instincts and a child's best interests disappeared [Rothman and Rothman, 1980, pp. 8–9].

3. The ownership conception of the parent-child relationship prevailed until the nineteenth century. Today, people still talk loosely of children belonging to parents. Yet, especially if we present hypothetical cases involving normal children, it is difficult to find consistent advocates of the proprietary view. Newborn children are not viewed as property the way (say) a pet could be. Pet owners are free to (painlessly) terminate the lives of an entire puppy litter if (for any reason whatever) they choose to do so. But no one would consider granting such rights to parents. Since we do not grant parents property rights over children, we cannot consistently argue that, when a defective child is born, the parents are the ones to decide its fate because "it belongs to them."

4. Surely the fact that the parents have very much at stake in the decision requires that no decision be made without their involvement or without their side being heard. At a minimum, the decision must be one that could be seen by them as having been decided fairly; this is especially important if it is one that is not favorable to them. Although a decision made without their involvement may be a good one, those making it would not be acting justly or treating them with due respect. As Seneca said: "He who decides anything with the other side unheard, may have reached a just decision, but is not himself just" (*Medea*, II. 199–200).

What follows is that the decision must not be made paternalistically by the medical staff without parental involvement. What does *not* follow from these considerations of fairness is that the decision-making authority should belong exclusively or even primarily to the parents. The principle of not deciding "with the other side unheard" is, as we have seen, a principle that protects the parents. But consistency requires that it also be applied in the direction of the defective newborn. It follows that some effective means to ensure that the child's interests are also given full weight is necessary.

Concern for the child's interests is very much the nurses' concern. Nurses who are directly responsible for the care of such defective children are in an ideal position to play a major role in providing such advocacy for the newborn. Exactly how this can be done will depend on the particular circumstances and will vary accordingly. That the most effective means for advocacy must be sought is the constant in each situation.

5. If the institution of the family is to be maintained as a primary social entity, we must make a presumption that parental authority is legitimate and not readily overridden. Were medical personnel and representatives of the state to interpose themselves whenever, in their judgment, parents were acting in ways that adversely affected their offspring, we would destroy the parent-child relationship. The family as an important and autonomous entity would be undermined. (Of course, it is possible that the destruction of the family as a primary institution would be a good thing. But for present purposes I think it is safe to assume the contrary.)

6. Intervention whenever authorities thought parental action adversely affected their offspring would also violate the autonomy of the parents. One fundamental way people express their autonomy is in the decisions they make concerning how to rear their children. If health professionals and representatives of the state can stand over their shoulders and step in whenever, in their judgment, they can do a better job than the parents, the parents have lost parenting as an avenue for expressing autonomy.

The presumptions of legitimate parental authority and autonomy entail a *hesitancy* to intrude but not an absolute prohibition. If parental action puts the child in clear and present danger—that is, if their action (or inaction) is clearly a threat to the child's life *and* fundamental well-being—the presumptions are set aside and intrusion is warranted. The right of the newborn to have its vital and most-basic interests protected is in conflict with the right of parental autonomy. Surely, in these clear cases of conflict, the child's interests must be given priority. Not only is the intrusion warranted, it is required. In cases in which the fundamental well-being of the child is not so clearly at issue (for example, given the child's condition, we just do not know whether continued existence or being allowed to die without further intervention is best for the child), the presumption of parental autonomy should prevail.

One final consideration on the issue of who should decide: if one party (e.g., the doctors or the parents) is given the exclusive right to decide moral questions and set policy in accordance with that choice, and if all others involved are expected to carry out the decisions, the other participants are vulnerable. They may be required to carry out actions they find morally repugnant. The nurses' plight in the Johns Hopkins case is a clear example. Having had no input into the decision, the nurses are told to provide professional nursing care to the newborn but not to feed it—for it has been brought to the nursery to die. (The routine, life-saving surgery that would have been insisted upon [if necessary, by going to the courts] had the child been normal was withheld from this infant because it was a victim of Down's syndrome.) Some have argued that the nurses should have refused to take on this assignment. One consideration that could be offered in support of refusal is that basic care such as changing, bathing, or holding prolongs the life of the infant. Care that prolongs the life of an infant who has been set aside to die of malnutrition is of questionable value—and arguably is not consistent with good nursing practice. Another consideration that supports refusal is that even if we were to agree that the parents have the moral right to decide whether to treat the child and that, therefore, we ought not to *prevent* them from making and carrying out their decision, it does not follow that anyone has a duty to *assist* them in carrying it out. The parents could take the child home and allow it to die, rather than have the nurses supervise its dying. In order for there to be cooperation, teamwork, and high morale, it is essential that all affected parties—including nurses—be full partners in the decision-making process. Nurses working with defective newborns should contribute to the efforts to increase the team practice approach.

Now we turn from the question of who should decide, to the question of what principles should guide the decisions whether to treat. Several principles are suggested in the following scenario:

The four-day-old infant was being maintained on a respirator due to severe respiratory deficiency. While there had not been time for chromosomal analysis, all evidence pointed to a diagnosis of a genetic disorder leading to severe mental retardation, growth failure, and numerous anatomical abnormalities (Trisomy 18). While there have been scattered reports of patients with the anomaly living to adulthood, 87% die within the first year of life.

A conference is being held to decide what to do with the infant.

The chief of pediatrics reported several conversations with the father who had said, "If you cannot guarantee that my child will be normal, I don't want you to do anything for it. I am not willing to raise an abnormal child." The chief said that he shared the feelings of the father and had told him, "I promise to do everything in my power to see that your wishes are carried out."

A psychiatrist also had several conversations with the father, and feels that the father is presently in a state of acute denial. If the respirator were turned off at the father's initiative, later guilt feelings could create psychiatric problems for him. He recommends that the respirator be turned off immediately but that the father be told simply that the child died despite the best care the medical team could provide.

The psychiatric social worker states that she feels that the family would be put under extreme stress if the infant were brought home.

A pediatric resident called attention to a patient of his own, who has a slight respiratory difficulty but cannot be put on a respirator because the Trisomy 18 infant is using the last available machine. Without the respirator, the other infant, who is otherwise healthy, may run a 50% risk of some brain damage.

At this point, the nurse who has been most directly responsible for the care of the infant interrupted. She insisted that the infant had every right to live and could not be allowed to die simply because it was not normal or was not wanted or was on a machine which could be beneficial to another [adapted from Brody, 1976, p. 101 and Veatch, 1977, pp. 36–37].

One of the principles implicit in the conference debate is that normalcy is a necessary condition for a life to be worth living. By whatever means (in this case deception), the medical team should shelter the family (here the father—the mother is not mentioned) from the full impact of their (the family's) decision to let the infant die. The burdens a defective child would bring to a family are relevant to a decision concerning whether to treat a defective newborn. In a situation of scarcity of medical resources (e.g., respirators) it is appropriate to displace a poor-prognosis infant in order to provide intensive care for a better-prognosis infant.

The nurse, acting as a client advocate of the infant, speaks against these principles: normalcy is not a necessary condition for the gift of life. The infant has a right or claim to life that cannot be overridden by considerations of hardship to others. And an infant already on a life-sustaining machine may not be removed from it because another would benefit more from it.

The principles involved in the debate, although rather vague and general, provide us with a good point of departure. If we consider the fact that a person could agree with the implicit principles espoused by the nurse and yet disagree with her about their meaning and how they should be applied to this case, we see the need for making them more precise. In order to work out a somewhat more-precise set of principles, let us consider the questions these principles are designed to answer:

1. What makes a life not worth living or such that death is to be preferred to the restricted life that is possible?

2. Is it ever right to withhold available life-saving therapy from a defective newborn?

3. Is it ever right to withdraw life-sustaining equipment from either a dying infant or one that is defective?

4. Is it ever right to withdraw life support (e.g., a respirator) from one infant to make it available to another having a better prognosis?

We shall consider these questions in order. 1. To say that normalcy is a necessary condition for a life to be worth living is extremely rigid and a contention, upon reflection, we are not likely to feel comfortable supporting. Too many people with serious handicaps and defects have lived lives that are an inspiration to us all. Examples such as Helen Keller and John Merrick (subject of the Broadway play and the movie *The Elephant Man*) immediately come to mind. These are, of course, the notable exceptions, but they show that normalcy is far too rigid and narrow a standard. One of the troubling aspects of the Down's syndrome case discussed earlier is that, although far from "normal," we feel very uneasy with the conclusion that death is a better alternative than life for the individual. Typically, the victims of the disease have an I.Q. range of 50 to 80, are trainable, can perform simple jobs, are of happy disposition, are capable of expressing love, and can live a long time.

The anencephalic infant (born without a developed brain) is one of the clearest examples of a human being having such a poor prognosis that probably most people would agree that its death would be a blessing. A baby suffering from anencephaly ordinarily is so severely retarded that it has virtually no prospect of ever gaining more than minimum control over bodily movements and functions. It has no chance of developing those traits that separate humans from other (lower) forms of animal life and endow humanity with dignity— namely, self-consciousness, autonomy, and rationality. Victims are not trainable or able to interact with others and express love. The potentiality for human relationships—the basis upon which a life of value and dignity can be lived—is missing. As Richard A. McCormick has said:

Life is not a value to be preserved in and for itself. . . . It is a value to be preserved precisely as a condition for other values, and therefore insofar as these other values remain attainable. Since these other values cluster around and are rooted in human relationships, it seems to follow that life is a value to be preserved only insofar as it contains some potentiality for human relationships [McCormick, 1974, p. 175].

In cases such as the anencephalic, respect for what is human about human life should restrain our intervention. To compel such a child to live when all that is of value is missing is not doing it a favor. From a value perspective, one is thereby sentencing the child to a fate worse than death.

The characteristics the anencephalic lacks but that an individual with Down's syndrome typically has point to the basic requirements of a life worth living or of sufficiently high quality to be preferable to nonexistence. The problematic cases are those that lie between. In each case (if possible) a determination must be made as to where on the continuum the case lies. Using the clear cases as guidance, one must determine how the case at hand compares. For example, cases of spina bifida (birth defects that involve an opening in the spine) fall at the various points along the continuum. Some of these will have prognoses more similar to the anencephalic and therefore will fall below the threshhold, whereas others will have prognoses comparable to that of Down's syndrome and thus are on the other side of the threshhold.

2. Our answer to the first question provides us with a basis for answering the second: whether it is ever right to withhold life-saving therapy from a defective newborn. We can see that our decision must depend on the severity of the defect. For the child whose condition places him below the threshhold, we can offer a justification for withholding the treatment that appeals to the best interests of the child. In such cases, if a child's life is prolonged by our efforts we are causing it injury. H. Tristram Engelhardt, Jr., has argued that prolonging lives of those infants whose condition places them below the threshhold is wrongfully to inflict life on them. It is to cause a "wrongful life." (For a discussion of the use of the notion of "wrongful life" in the law, see Creighton, 1977.) Engelhardt bases him claim on the following premises: (a) medicine now can cause the prolongation of the life of seriously deformed children who in the past would have died young; (b) it is not clear that life so prolonged is a good for the child; further, (c) the choice is made not on the basis of costs to the parents or to society but on the basis of the child's suffering and compromised existence (Engelhardt, 1975).

Engelhardt offers examples of infants who should not be treated, in accordance with this line of reasoning:

In the case of Tay-Sachs disease (a disease marked by a progressive increase in spasticity and dementia usually leading to death at age three or four), one can hardly imagine that the terminal stages of spastic reaction to stimuli and great difficulty in swallowing are at all pleasant to the child (even insofar as it can only minimally perceive its circumstances). If such a child develops aspiration pneumonia and is treated, it can reasonably be said that to prolong its life is to inflict suffering. Other diseases give fairly clear portraits of lives not worth living: for example, Lesch-Nyham disease, which is marked by mental retardation and compulsive self-mutation [Engelhardt, 1975, pp. 187–88].

The report of an interdisciplinary conference convened to consider the ethical problems raised by neonatal intensive care concisely states the conclusion we have argued here: "Life-preserving intervention should be understood as doing harm to an infant who cannot survive infancy, or will live in intractible pain, or cannot participate even minimally in human experience" (Jonsen, et. al., 1975, p. 760).

3. Often people feel there is an important difference between withholding life-saving therapy and withdrawing such therapy. Sometimes the former is seen as passive or as an act of omission, while the latter is seen as active or as an act of commission. In many contexts, including this one, acts of commission are felt to require more stringent justification than acts of omission. Following this line of reasoning, support beyond what was given above for sometimes withholding life-sustaining therapy is required to defend decisions to withdraw it.

The commonly held assumptions that there is a moral difference between active and passive termination of life and that withdrawing treatment (e.g., turning off a respirator) is active as opposed to passive must be examined. This we shall do in the next section concerning the treatment of the terminally ill.

The question whether it is ever right to withdraw life-sustaining equipment from a dying infant can be answered without determining the correctness of these assumptions. Consider the following case:

A 32-year-old gave premature birth during the thirty-second week of pregnancy to a 1600-gram boy. The baby showed evidence of hyaline membrane disease and was placed on a respirator the second day after birth. Vital signs were present, although there was some difficulty in respiration. The infant was on the respirator for forty-five days, after which time he showed no evidence of 0_2 toxicity and was taken off the respirator. At that point PO_2 levels were within the normal range, all neurological signs were normal, and there was a normal EEG, but continued evidence of respiratory difficulty resulted in a decision to return the infant to the respirator. At two-and-a-half months there was evidence of congestive heart failure, which was treated with digitalis. There were noticeable changes in the neurological picture, including definite evidence of deterioration. Over the next several weeks attempts to wean the infant from the respirator failed. At four-and-a-half months, there were definite signs of brain damage and no hope of improvement in respiration. The physicians, in consultation with the nurses, other medical staff, and the parents, decided to take the infant off the respirator and they agreed not to resuscitate in the nearly certain and imminent event of respiratory arrest [adapted from a case presented by Veatch, 1977, p. 333].

In deciding what course of action is morally justified, we must question, as Robert Veatch does, whether continuation of treatment after steady and progressive deterioration and signs of brain damage is saving his life or "merely having his death prolonged" (Veatch, 1977, p. 338). In cases such as this, continued intervention is more likely to be done for the benefit of others than for the infant. The medical intervention is the cause of continued existence, but continued existence, in a case such as this, is an injury, a prolongation of suffering. The duty not to injure the infant requires discontinuing the intervention, knowing that death is likely to ensue.

The issues introduced in these final paragraphs will be developed systematically in the next section on the nurse and the terminally ill client. Modern medical technology has brought us so much that can contribute to living better, fuller, and longer lives. But the more awesome responsibilities that this new power gives us is nowhere more evident than in decisions that must now be made concerning the care of the terminally ill.

Finally, the last of the four questions raised by the debate over how to treat the Trisomy 18 infant (if it is ever right to withdraw life support from one child to make it available to another) has not been discussed. It too is being deferred to a later discussion, the chapter on justice (Chapter 8). The reason for this is that the issue is best addressed after we have had the opportunity to consider several general and theoretical points about the fair distribution of scarce life-saving medical resources.

The Nurse and the Dying Patient

The problem of proper care for the dying is an age-old one. In Plato's *Republic,* written in ancient Greece, Socrates praises a physician who acted on the policy that "bodies which disease had penetrated through and through he would not have attempted to cure . . . He did not want to lengthen out good-for-nothing lives" (*Republic,* III, 407c). The questions of this chapter are perennial ones: How can we make dying more gentle and humane? Do we have a right willingly to embrace death, either for ourselves or for others?

What gives these questions a new urgency is our increased capacity to sustain life beyond reasonable hope of recovery. Medical technology such as respirators, heart-lung machines, and intravenous feeding make it possible for us to keep a person alive for long periods of time with little, if any, prospect for recovery or even for regaining consciousness. These capabilities force us to consider: When is our striving to keep others alive no longer "helping" them? The highly publicized, tragic case of Karen Quinlan, a young woman maintained for months on a respirator after prolonged respiratory arrest produced irreversible brain damage, has become a symbol of this concern and a catalyst for discussion and even legislative action concerning the proper treatment of the dying.

In addition to making the problem more urgent, medical and other technological advances have changed the common causes and mode of dying. Before the advent of modern medicine, death was likely to be caused by infectious disease. Death was neither as unexpected nor as drawn out as is frequently the case today. Instead of a hospital bed, one was more likely to die in one's own bed, surrounded by family and friends.

Today, accidents, homicide and suicide are the principal causes of death among young people, and chronic diseases are the principal causes of death among the old. Furthermore, it is now highly probable that when a person dies, his death will be either sudden and unexpected, as in an accident, or else long and drawn out, with pain and mental or physical deterioration. In the latter case, more than likely it will be in a hospital bed rather than at home [Ladd, 1979, p. 4].

Jeanne Quint, in *The Nurse and the Dying Patient*, has stated more specifically how death typically comes to patients under contemporary nurses' care:

Obviously the unexpected death can happen anywhere, but in the hospital certain types of death tend to be associated with certain ward settings. The emergency room deals with violent death brought in from the community. In the operating room a prearranged treatment may go awry and cause sudden death. In medical and surgical wards death not uncommonly appears after a progressive downhill course, which may be rapid or prolonged [Quint, 1967, p. 117].

Another nurse, Mary Chudleigh, has provided a general description of the nurses' role in this context.

Dealing with the dying on their deathbed is one facet of caring for the dying; the most taxing role for the nurse is in caring for individuals between the time they are first diagnosed and the time they will be really terminal; years may elapse. The nurse's position in caring for the dying is very human. Nurses must care about people if they are to function well in this setting. It is emotionally exhausting [Chudleigh, 1978, p. 244].

In the modern hospital, the nurse more than any other health professional is likely to develop a close relationship with the client and be in a strong position to judge the needs and wishes of the client as a person, a special individual.

Nursing provides continuous twenty-four-hour-a-day monitoring of the institutionalized patient. The duties of a nurse are intrusive; there is no way to avoid personal contact of this sort without emotional involvement. The act of bathing patients, feeding them or just seeing that they are eating enough, changing the bed when it's dirty, monitoring equipment to make sure its functioning, making sure intake and output are adequate and balanced, just these physical duties bring the nurse and patient into a close interpersonal relationship. Because of this relationship, the nurse is usually the one to explain what the physician really says: the prognosis is poor with a six-month life expectancy [Chudleigh, 1978, pp. 249–50].

For the dying person who is beyond medical help (the "hopeless patient"), nursing care is what offers the client the chance to live out his or her days with as much dignity and comfort as possible. As Cleary says in "The Nurse and the Dying Patient":

The nurse has traditionally been the health professional most central to patients and families confronted with imminent death. In hospitals and nursing homes the nurse is involved in the personal care of the terminally ill; community-based public health nurses and visiting nurse services attempt to assist the dying at home. The focus of nursing care is comfort and reassurance for families and the use of therapeutic skills to maintain body integrity and functioning for the patient [Cleary, 1978, p. 177].

In the root meaning of the word, the nurse is concerned with euthanasia—which in Greek means "a good death." Today, of course, the meaning has changed to that of "mercy killing." Much of the discussion concerning care for the dying has focused on justifications for mercy killing. What is unfortunate about this is that the fundamental issues concerning care for the dying—namely, what we ought to do to improve the quality of the remaining life and to make dying more gentle and humane—tend to become lost in a thicket of distinctions and, in some cases, sophistry.

The hospice movement is a shining example of people conscientiously and directly dealing with these basic issues in the care of dying. As we discussed in an earlier chapter, the hospice is essentially a nursing care concept in which nurses function as the major providers and coordinators of client care.

The hospice is a concept derived from ancient times, connoting a place where travelers, pilgrims, the sick, wounded, or dying could find rest and comfort. Its contemporary meaning implies a program of care offered to people completing their journey through life—a way station for the terminally ill. The philosophy of the hospice is provision of palliative and supportive care to dying patients and to their families, with emphasis on symptom control and preparation for and support during and after death. The aim of hospice programs is to improve the quality of the remaining life [Cleary, 1978, p. 197].

This is not the place to go into the details of hospice care. Suffice it to say that there are various types of hospice programs: from separate facilites designed exclusively for care of the dying, to special units within the general hospital in which nursing care consistent with the hospice concept is provided, to symptom control teams who are available for consultation (Cleary, 1978, pp. 197–98; see also Paige and Looney, 1977). Whatever the specific institutional framework, the aim of these efforts is to help terminally ill clients meet death without pain and under the most normal circumstances possible.

Had we begun with the ethical theory outlined in chapter one and asked what fundamental aim ought a nurse to have in dealing with the terminally ill, we would have to come to the same result. If we wish to honor clients' autonomy and respect their rights to determine as much as possible the direction their lives shall take, then our basic concern will be to interfere as little as possible with the life-style, habits, and patterns of living of the terminally ill while providing the means and assistance necessary for them to be able to exercise their choice. Hence, we would work to establish and maintain the most normal (for that client) circumstances possible, providing, for example, a cheerful environment in which "comfort and compassion are the guiding precepts" (Cleary, 1978, p. 197). Since, for most people, pain is debilitating and saps one's energy and initiative (and, hence, is an enemy of self-determination), we would work to minimize pain without reducing lucidity. If a trade-off had to be made between a longer life—but with pain and in far from normal settings (e.g., on many monitors in intensive care)—and a somewhat shorter life—but with minimal pain and in more normal circumstances (perhaps even the client's home)—we would allow the client to choose the shorter life. Extending a client's life for as long as possible is a reasonable goal for medical treatment; but it does not take precedence over the nurse's (and physician's) most fundamental moral objective, namely, helping the client to exercise his or her autonomy and treating him or her as a person. In case of conflict, we must opt for the latter.

In the literature on care of the dying, much of the discussion focuses on the choice of prolonged life in great pain, on the one hand, or, on the other, either of two possibilities: analgesic dosages that relieve the pain but also risk shortening the client's life, or the "merciful overdose" which simply ends the life as well as the suffering. Dramatic accounts abound of situations that appear to force us to make this choice. Stewart Alsop (a well-known journalist), when he himself was dying of a rare form of cancer in 1975, wrote the following account of a terminally ill client he called Jack, with whom he shared a room:

The third night that I roomed with Jack in our tiny double room in the solid-tumor ward of the cancer clinic of the National Institutes of Health in Bethesda, Md., a terrible thought occurred to me.

Jack had a melanoma in his belly, a malignant solid tumor that the doctors guessed was about the size of a softball. The cancer had started a few months before with a small tumor in his left shoulder, and there had been several operations since. The doctors planned to remove the softball-sized tumor, but they knew Jack would soon die. The cancer had metastasized—it had spread beyond control.

Jack was good-looking, about 28, and brave. He was in constant pain, and his doctor had prescribed an intravenous shot of a synthetic opiate—a pain-killer, or analgesic—every four hours. His wife spent many of the daylight hours with him, and she would sit or lie on his bed and pat him all over, as one pats a child, only more methodically, and this seemed to help control the pain. But at night, when his pretty wife had left (wives cannot stay overnight at the NIH clinic) and darkness fell, the pain would attack without pity.

At the prescribed hour, a nurse would give Jack a shot of the synthetic analgesic, and this would control the pain for perhaps two hours or a bit more. Then he would begin to moan, or whimper, very low, as though he didn't want to wake me. Then he would begin to howl, like a dog.

When this happened, either he or I would ring for a nurse, and ask for a pain-killer. She would give him some codeine or the like by mouth, but it never did any real good—it affected him no more than half an aspirin might affect a man who had just broken his arm. Always the nurse would explain as encouragingly as she could that there was not long to go before the next intravenous shot—"Only about 50 minutes now." And always poor Jack's whimpers and howls would become more loud and frequent until at last the blessed relief came.

The third night of this routine, the terrible thought occurred to me. "If Jack were a dog," I thought, "what would be done with him?" The answer was obvious: the pound, and chloroform. No human being with a spark of pity could let a living thing suffer so, to no good end [Alsop, 1971].

If we are forced to make a choice between Jack's continued life of agony or mercifully ending it, (with Alsop) our humanity cries out: enough of this pointless suffering, let mercy triumph. Given his bleak prognosis and his intense suffering, Jack is beyond harm. Life holds nothing but torment. Death would be a release from bondage. And—if Jack requested it—death would in no way deprive him of that which he wants or violate his right to life. (If a person asks to be killed, the killing is not a violation of indivdual rights. If it is wrong, it is wrong for some other reason.)

Nevertheless, before we take the path of justifying active killing or some passive form of hastening death (in cases such as this), we must ask whether the only options are a life of pain or mercifully ending the client's life. Cecily Saunders, the founder of the famous St. Christopher's Hospice in England, maintains that pain and suffering can virtually always be controlled by the proper use of painkilling drugs and sleep-inducing medication (Saunders, 1973, pp. 30–31). Cleary, writing on hospices in 1978, claims that medication is available that both allows the client to be free of pain and to be mentally alert and able to participate in meaningful activities and relationships (Cleary, 1978, pp. 197–98). Others, too, have claimed that modern methods of overcoming pain are effective and can relieve the pain without hastening death (cf. Veatch, 1976, p. 94). If these claims are correct, then in Jack's case there likely was a third alternative which has the advantages of each without their disadvantages—continued existence relatively free from pain.

If such a third alternative is available, the empirical assumptions are false upon which arguments for hastening death or actively killing are often based. From a moral point of view, we can see the importance of considering whether all the alternatives have been explored. Of the alternatives we think are available, we may have chosen the best. Yet our choice is the wrong one, for we have failed to consider another available alternative that is superior. The third alternative, which is frequently not considered in discussions of treatment of dying clients, shows greatest respect for the client as a person. If only two choices were available, those advocating some form of hastening death might be right. But whenever a client's pain can be controlled, the superiority of this third alternative makes mercifully ending the client's life morally unacceptable.

Since one of the special skills of the nurse is pain control, the nurse has a major contribution to make in seeing to it that continued existence relatively free from pain is possible for more and more clients. We have seen the contribution nurses have already made. The opportunities for continued and increasing impact on the humane care of the dying must not be lost.

One of the greatest fears of mankind through the ages has been that of the fear of death. This fear may be of death itself or of what comes after death (e.g., eternal punishment). It may be of the "event" of dying. Nursing, with its holistic, compassionate concern for the dying person, must be directed at helping the client handle this fear.

If it is fear of death itself, the nurse will want to assist the client by seeing to it that, if desired, spiritual counseling is available. If it is the "event" of death (dying) that is feared, however, this is the immediate concern of physicians and nurses. The fear of dying may be a fear of the pain that the client anticipates. Obviously, if (as in hospice care) the client can be reassured that any accompanying pain can be controlled, much will have been done to allay these fears.

Often a client's fear of dying is the fear of abandonment, the fear of dying alone. An approach such as hospice care minimizes these fears. Family, friends, and volunteers, as well as nurses, are able to be with the dying client in surroundings that are as comfortable as possible. Staff who themselves are willing to accept the fact of death will be less prone to ignore or avoid the dying client. (Frequently cited in the literature on care of the dying is the fact that health professionals, usually nurses, tend to respond less quickly to the call from a dying client than from others.)

The fear of dying may also be a fear of a loss of dignity, of being treated as an object and even as a nuisance. Clearly, an approach to the dying client following the hospice model also minimizes these fears. When the needs of the person as a person are lost sight of and only the disease is treated (as can so easily and understandably happen in intensive care units), the client has good reason to fear for his or her dignity.

In order to consider the complex issues surrounding the question of the ethical care of the dying from the perspective adopted in Chapter 1, we have begun this discussion with a consideration of care of dying clients who are relatively free of pain and who are conscious and competent. Discussions of proper care for the dying frequently start at the other end, with the terminally ill client who is in intractible pain, or is comatose, or is incompetent. To do this is dangerous, however, because the focus then tends to be on medical decision-making concerning the client, rather than on the client's own wishes and interests. The fundamental requirement of respect for persons and their autonomy gets shunted to a secondary role. Yet, any discussion of the nurse and the dying client must address the cases of terminally ill clients whose pain cannot be controlled, terminally ill clients in a coma, and terminally ill clients who for one reason or another (e.g., senility) are judged to be incompetent. We do so now with our discussion of treatment of the conscious, competent client as our point of departure.

Because our fundamental moral concern is to preserve the client's autonomy, we must encourage people to express their views about the kinds of treatment they would want should they lapse into incompetency or a coma. One method of doing this is the "living will," a document expressing one's choices concerning terminal care which a client can sign while healthy. It states:

Death is as much a reality as birth, growth, maturity and old age—it is the one certainty of life. If the time comes when I, _____ can no longer take part in decisions for my own future, let this statement stand as an expression of my wishes, while I am still of sound mind.

If the situation should arise in which there is no reasonable expectation of my recovery from physical or mental disability, I request that I be allowed to die and not be kept alive by artifical means or "heroic measures." I do not fear death itself as much as the indignities of deterioration, dependence and hopeless pain. I, therefore, ask that medication be mercifully administered to me to alleviate suffering even though this may hasten the moment of death. [A Euthanasia Education Council publication]

The "living will" makes clear that the locus of choice lies with the dying person. It is a powerful expression of client autonomy. Yet it has some clear limitations. Although helpful in giving some guidance and in protecting a client's freedom of choice, obviously the document is (of necessity) too vague to cover all contingencies. Another concern is that a person's views could change after the document is signed. This possibility undermines confidence others can have that it truly is an expression of that person's views. Despite these limitations, for the person whose concern is to have some say about his or her own death, even a vague and legally nonbinding document is better than nothing.

Of course, if the living will could be improved upon, that would be better. To that end, instruments other than the living will have been prepared. One of the more promising means of ensuring that care be consistent with one's own desires and interests when one cannot express them oneself is to give someone—a spouse, relative, friend, or lawyer—power of attorney. As one's agent, this person can speak for the client who is incapable of exercising his or her own judgment. This also is by no means foolproof. But such strategies offer great promise in the struggle to maintain client autonomy.

Besides client responsibility to make their wishes known (by means of instruments such as the living will or through the power of attorney), health professionals have a responsibility to make every reasonable effort to know the client's wishes. This is a prerequisite for performing the task of promoting client autonomy. Knowing these wishes, the health professional has a *prima facie* duty to honor them; i.e., the client's wishes concerning treatment must be honored unless there is some other more compelling obligation the fulfillment of which conflicts with doing so. (In Chapter 5, we shall examine some of the fundamental obligations that may come into conflict.)

Consider the following case, which raises the issue of honoring a client's wishes:

A patient in the cardiac unit who was admitted with a massive myocardial infarction begins to show signs of increased cardiac failure. The patient and the family have clearly expressed their desire to the medical and nursing staff to refrain from "heroics" should complications arise. The patient stops breathing and the intern begins to intubate the patient, requests the nurses's assistance, and orders a respirator [Mappes, 1981, p. 99].

In this case, let us stipulate that the nurse is aware of the client's wishes, whereas the intern is not. Surely the nurse would be obliged to inform the intern of the client's clearly stated wishes that the staff refrain from such procedures. Assuming the intern also wishes to honor the client's autonomy, he or she would then have reason not to proceed. (If the intern refuses, we have a classic example of a nurse-physician conflict as discussed in Chapter 3.) Were the nurse to fail to inform the intern, clearly the client's autonomy would not be respected.

What ought to be done in this case is quite clear because it does not present us with conflicting obligations that could outweigh the duty to honor the client's wishes. Whether or not one shares the view that client autonomy should be one's most fundamental commitment, those who reflect on this case are likely to agree that the right thing to do is to refrain from efforts to resuscitate, thereby honoring the client's request.

In many other cases, however, it may seem equally clear that the client's wishes concerning terminal treatment should *not* be honored. Suppose, for example, that a terminal client begs for an overdose of morphine. Another client requests that the support systems keeping him alive be removed. In these cases we may not be sure that we should acquiesce in their wishes. Should not other duties be given priority here? For example, doesn't the generally accepted prohibition against taking the life of a human being for any reason other than self-defense (and, possibly, war and capital punishment) take priority over any duties to respect a person's autonomy?

In Chapter 5 we shall discuss paternalism—acting in ways that go against a person's own immediate desires or wishes in order to protect or advance the "true" interests of the person. As we shall see, under certain conditions, we may feel we ought to do so. We may judge that the client is not competent and, hence, we ought not to act in accordance with his or her wishes, but rather in accordance with what seems to us to be his or her best interests. In other cases (these are the ones we are discussing in this chapter) we may feel that the client's request would violate fundamental moral principles (in particular, that one ought not to take another's life) and so ought not to be honored.

The status of the prohibition against killing must be addressed if we are going to come to terms with how to treat the terminally ill. We could make the prohibition against killing an absolute and fundamental principle in our ethical theory. Sometimes those who speak of the sanctity of human life have such a view in mind. In contrast, the position developed in this chapter considers the prohibition against taking human life to be derivative from the fundamental principle of respect for persons and the duty to refrain from harming another, as developed in Chapter 1. Respect for oneself and others as rational creatures is incompatible with holding life cheaply and being willing to terminate life lightly. In most cases, a person values his or her life, and thus respect for that person requires that we not interfere with that person's autonomy. Killing him or her is the most dramatic type of infringement. Nonetheless, this reasoning does not apply in cases in which the person does not value his or her life due (say) to illness or injury that has resulted in the loss of genuinely human life before biological death. If one were to comply with his or her request, no right to life is being infringed. The person has requested that his or her life be ended. He or she has "waived" the right. Complying with the request by no means indicates that life is being viewed as cheap (being willing casually to dispense with it). Nor in these cases can we object that death causes *harm* to the individual. The person is "beyond injury" (Brandt, 1975). Hence, taking another's life is not necessarily impermissible; the prohibition is not an absolute one.

Another argument that has been advanced to establish the absolute prohibition against causing another's death is that it follows from the health professional's professional role. For example, some maintain that a physician's primary duty is to save lives. No other duty can ever take priority over this. If such a position could be defended, it would follow that the physician would never be justified in acting to terminate a client's life. Of course, whether saving lives is (in every case) the overriding duty of the physician is debatable. Alleviating suffering and promoting health certainly are also duties of the physician. Is it necessarily the case that these must always take second place to saving lives? This seems unlikely. To answer this for the physician, however, we would have to consider the physician's role as we did the nurse's role in Chapter 2. From the discussion of the nurse's role we can see that saving lives is *not* the highest or an absolute professional duty of the nurse. As a client advocate, the nurse's fundamental duty is to promote and defend the client's choices and interests. The professional duty to save lives is derived from this basic duty. So an argument appealing to professional role does not yield the conclusion that the nurse's duty to refrain from taking a life *must* be given priority.

If an appeal to professional role does not yield the conclusion that the duty to refrain from taking a life must be given priority over clients' wishes and best interests, it may yield a weaker conclusion: that the professional is never obligated to take action or refrain from action that leads to a client's death. Consider the following two cases, one of refraining from acting, which results in the client's death, and the other of taking action that leads to the client's death:

(A)

One evening I came on just as this patient came in. She was 50 years old and she was 50 percent burned. In ten minutes I loved this lady. They had just gotten through admitting her, debriding her, tanking her [pulling off dead skin and washing her in a whirlpool].

When I went into the room and met this lady, I couldn't believe how alert and cheerful she was. It didn't even seem like scared cover-up. She was great. She was probably in shock. She told me how it had happened and that it was really an accident—with burns sometimes it's hard to tell. I left the room after about ten minutes and she seemed supercontent.

An hour later I went back in to take her vital signs; I couldn't believe it—dead. I was so shocked because I had just left this lady talking and smiling.

I went out to the lounge and said to the doctor, "She's dead."

"Who's dead?" he asked me. We weren't expecting anyone to die right then. I said, "The lady you just admitted." He jumped up and raced out of there like a bat out of hell. Got to her door and stopped cold.

"What should I do?" he asked me. He was the resident.

"You going to pound on her chest?" I asked. "She's cold. I mean she's dead. What are you going to do? Is she going to live anyway?"

He went running at first as though he were Superman, and then he stopped short at the door and all he said was "What should I do?" He stood outside where he couldn't see the patient.

The discussion that followed wasn't between us. It was inside each of us. Individual. He was fighting with himself. "I hate to pronounce anybody dead," he said, looking at me. "It feels like such a final thing," and, still not going into the room, "I always think, What if? God forbid."

I looked in the room and looked at him. Her monitor was a flat line, flat as a board. I said, "I think she's dead."

After several minutes, he finally went in to pronounce her dead, and I stood there going over what had happened. I had walked in, seen her, slapped her, and checked her pulse. Nothing. I was so shocked, I didn't expect it. I wasn't prepared. . . . I decided not to call a code. I had images of the woman laughing with me just a half hour before. So it took me a minute or so to check, and then I remembered the doctor saying, "Her spirits are good, but I still don't think she'll make it. But. . . "

I walked out of there very slowly, taking my time before I told the doctor. I don't know exactly the moment, but I know I decided not to try to bring her back. I really was crazy about her. There would have been so much pain, and there was practically no chance that she would have survived the burns [Daniels, 1979, p. 40].

(B)

Sandy was a five-year-old kid. I had been taking care of her for several months. She had a malignant brain tumor. They had operated several times, her head was shaved, and she had scars like zippers over her head. She got worse and worse and finally slipped into a coma. Her parents used to be at the hospital every day; they'd take turns minding Sandy's twin brothers, who were three years old. The mother couldn't stand it and finally took a bunch of sleeping pills. The doctors used to stand at the foot of the bed and shake their heads saying, "Medicine can't do any more." The mother survived the pills and after that she used to talk to me. One night, Sandy just stopped breathing and would you believe some nut jumped on her chest and her heart started beating again. They put her on a respirator. She got infected and then the doctors started giving her antibiotics, sticking her with needles all the time. The kid looked like a pincushion. She was getting all black-and-blue, and nothing seemed to touch the infection. She smelled awful. Sort of pungent and sickly sweet, like decaying tissue. I could even smell it when I was out of the room. It stuck in my nostrils, and if I breathed through my mouth I could taste it. My clothes and hair and skin smelled like it too.

She had been such a pretty little girl, and I really cared about her. I kept asking everyone how we could get her off that damn machine. Nobody could do it . . . although they all agreed it would be better if she died. They told me if her heart stopped again to walk slow before I called anyone. I knew what they meant. Her father came in one day and told me he couldn't stand it anymore. He was going to run as far away as he could get. I thought about the twins and about the mother. Sandy had died once.

I went into her room to bathe her as I always did, and this time I closed the door. I took her off. Then I bathed her and powdered her and fixed her bed. By the time I hooked her up again, her heart had stopped. . . . As soon as I took her off, I could breathe better [Daniels, 1979, p.41].

It seems to me that what the nurses did in these two cases is praiseworthy. Their actions were morally justifiable and commendable. To say this, however, is very different from saying that what they did was morally *obligatory*. They have gone beyond the call of duty—beyond their legal duty as nurses and their moral duty as client advocates. The response of nurses who, when asked what they thought about mercy killing, said: "I could only do it for someone I loved," is a correct moral as well as personal response. Active killing, if justified in these cases, is an act of charity rather than a performance of duty.

From the various cases cited and our discussion of them, we can derive the following set of principles:

1. The nurse is *obliged* to honor the competent client's wishes insofar as this entails refraining from actions the client has explicitly stated he or she did not want done. Failure to meet this obligation would be incompatible with both the principle of autonomy and the concept of the nurse as client advocate.

2. The nurse does not have an obligation to *assist* the client in his or

her desire to die. An obligation to assist in this way does not follow from the autonomy principle. (The analogy of the right to free speech discussed earlier can be used as the model here. I infringe upon your right to free speech if I interfere with your attempt to speak (e.g., shout you down or gag you). I would not be violating your free speech, however, were I to fail (or refuse) to help you to deliver a speech. My fundamental duty as a client advocate is to protect my clients' autonomy, that is, to prevent harm and unwarranted interference. We have seen from an examination of several cases that the nurse's duty to assist the client does not extend to assistance in dying. Yet in select cases (as in the examples just discussed), assisting the client may be morally commendable—an act of love going beyond the requirements of duty.

3. In cases in which the client's wishes have not been made clear or cannot be made clear, and death appears to objective observers to be the alternative that clearly is in the best interest of the client, the nurse has an obligation to prevent the initiation of procedures that prolong the client's dying. This follows from the protective role that a nurse as client advocate is called upon to play.

The points at which lines will be drawn following these principles correspond rather closely to those suggested by most other ethical theories when they are applied to issues in health care. Nevertheless, adherents of other theories, and especially adherents of the natural law theory, use several well-known and often-cited distinctions we have not mentioned. It is instructive to look at several of these distinctions.

According to natural law ethics, we are required to exercise all "ordinary" means to preserve a life. But "extraordinary" means need not be taken. By ordinary is meant all medicines, treatments, and operations that offer a reasonable hope of benefit for the patient and that can be obtained and used without excessive expense, pain, or other inconvenience. Extraordinary means are those that offer the client no reasonable hope and whose use involves serious hardships for the client or others. (Sometimes the ordinary-extraordinary means distinction is used to contrast standard or orthodox medical procedures from untried or experimental ones. This is quite a different meaning and not the meaning of these terms within the natural law tradition.)

If the only way a life can be prolonged is by extraordinary means, the client is morally permitted to refuse them and health professionals need not provide them. Extraordinary treatments also may be stopped on the dying. Ordinary means, however, may not be stopped nor may one, on this view, actively bring about a client's death (for example, by giving an overdose of a painkiller) *with the intention* of bringing about death. In contrast, if one's intention in giving the painkiller were to decrease the client's acute pain and an *unintended but foreseen* consequence of doing so is the hastening of his death, performing the action with its "double effect" is acceptable (according to natural law theorists).

The major difficulty with the extraordinary-ordinary means distinction is not that it attempts to draw the line in the wrong place; instead, the real difficulty comes in trying to apply its very vague criteria. When, for example, is the expense, pain or other inconvenience excessive? The same treatment in similar situations will appear excessively expensive or inconvenient to some and not to others. For example, the surgery to correct complications arising from spina bifida in a newborn suffering from this defect will be called extraordinary means by some, because in comparing the costs (expense, pain or other inconvenience) of the treatment with the advantages to be gained the costs seem excessive. Others will argue that such surgery is an ordinary means and, therefore, it is required no matter what the cost. What tends to happen is that the labels "ordinary" and "extraordinary" are applied, respectively, to treatments we consider binding or not binding. The actual decision concerning the appropriateness of the treatment is made on other grounds—for example, a straightforward utilitarian calculation of the cost-benefit ratio. Although proponents of the natural law view are (quite correctly) opposed to utilitarian-based decisions, the usual formulation of the ordinary-extraordinary distinction comes close to being just that, a disguised utilitarianism.

Instead of employing the ordinary-extraordinary means distinction, I have argued that these decisions can be made more effectively by using the criteria outlined above. Yet if we wish to *label* as extraordinary all treatments that dying clients reject or would reject because they merely prolong dying, no harm is done.

Another feature of the natural law theory is the importance placed on the intention of the nurse or doctor. If the intention of treatment that leads to a client's death is palliative and death is a foreseen but unintended byproduct, the action is morally defensible. If the treatment were intended to hasten the dying process, however, the action could not be condoned.

This distinction between direct and indirect action is a clear and understandable one. Yet it is unhelpful because of the difficulty of applying it in precisely those cases in which we are puzzled as to what we may do—those times we are most in need of a guiding principle. Consider, for example, the following cases in which it seems arbitrary to say either that the intention is to alleviate pain knowing (but not intending) that death will result, or that the intention is the death of the client (because of a desire to prevent continued suffering).

In a situation where potassium is routinely added to IV solution, if the nurse says to the doctor, "This patient's potassium is already high enough to almost stop his heart," and he answers, "Please don't do any more blood studies," and then, "He's terminal, you know," he means that a stopped heart is an easier death than being eaten away by cancer. If she agrees, she adds potassium as ordered and cancels the studies. If she doesn't agree, she refuses and lives with her patient's pain or asks another nurse to do it [Daniels, 1979, p. 38].

If we feel that a client's death may never be intended, this is because we consider death as *always* an evil or an injury. We have been arguing that death is not always such. If this is so, then in those cases there is no reason to insist that one may not intend the death of another. One need not make fine (sophistic?) distinctions to avoid admitting intending what we recognized as the preferred option (i.e., the best alternative among those available or the lesser of the several evils).

Often it is helpful to draw the distinction between what is intended, on the one hand, and what is foreseen as a consequence of one's actions but not intended, on the other. For example, an employer hires B rather than A or C, knowing that this will cause deep disappointment for both A and C. In choosing B she is *not* intending A's or C's disappointment. Similarly it is possible to increase a client's narcotic dosage, intending to relieve pain while knowing, although not intending, that this will cause respiratory depression and death. Nevertheless, in many cases (as in the case cited above) honesty may require us to admit that it is not altogether clear that we are not also intending the client's death or that separating the different ("double") effects is artificial and only a rationalization. I have argued that we do not need the rationalization. When conditions such as we have discussed hold, intending a client's death is morally defensible.

If acting with the intention of ending a client's life can be morally defended, one of the strongest (nontheological) reasons for an absolute prohibition against active (voluntary) euthanasia (i.e., deliberately killing a terminally ill client who has requested it) is removed. Still, there remain several important considerations which in many cases would tip the balance in favor of passive rather than active euthanasia. Consider cases in which there is the probability of an incorrect (too pessimistic) prediction concerning the course of the disease or a wrong diagnosis (e.g., the patient's condition is not hopeless). With passive euthanasia it may still be possible to detect and correct the mistakes, whereas in active euthanasia this would not be so. Obviously we would have to be certain of both the diagnosis and prognosis as well as the client's true wishes before active euthanasia could be condoned.

Were a policy of active euthanasia to be contemplated in cases in which the client has not requested it (nonvoluntary euthanasia), we would find that the potential for abuse and for disregarding the client's autonomy is too great to overcome possible benefit in the reduction of suffering and the indignity of prolonged dying that may result from having such a policy. Given the dangers, no one could feel secure with such a policy. It could not protect us from the possibility that terminally ill people would be killed to gain access to an inheritance, to free a hospital bed, to dispose of someone having no social value, or simply to get rid of an obstreperous client. In short, death could be chosen for reasons other than concern for the client (the only legitimate reason) and in ways that fail to respect the client's right to self-determination.

These are sufficient reasons for rejecting a *policy* of active euthanasia. Contrary to what may appear to follow, however, taking a stance against a policy of active euthanasia does not require us to continue treatment should the client no longer want it or should treatment no longer be serving any function other than prolonging dying. We have argued above that a procedure need not be started if a client refuses it or if it would simply prolong the process of dying when there is no hope of reversal. The same reasons apply to discontinuing treatment as for not beginning it. If one of these actions is right, so is the other. Given that not beginning treatment is acceptable in the situations cited, we can conclude that discontinuing it in these situations is morally acceptable as well.

Often the question of the justification of discontinuing treatment is dealt with on the terminological level. The participants appear to believe that the crucial issue is whether removal of life-support systems (e.g., a respirator) is active or passive killing. The question is difficult to resolve because this distinction is notoriously slippery. On the position developed in this chapter, however, the morality of the action in no way depends on our ability to classify it. If the client's informed, uncoerced request not to have certain actions performed is a sufficient reason not to begin a treatment, it would also be sufficient for discontinuing a treatment. The refusal of additional treatment removes the duty to continue what has been started. Similarly, if we agree that there is no obligation to put a client on a respirator when that would merely prolong his or her dying, then—if similar reasons obtain for disconnecting the respirator (i.e., continuation merely prolongs dying)—there is no obligation to continue it. Of course, psychologically there would be a difference. Carrying out the decision not to put a client on a respirator, for example, normally would be far less traumatic than would be carrying out the decision to turn off the machine after someone had been on it for a time.

Related to, but clearly distinct from, the question of when to stop treatment is the question of when death occurs. This is a complex issue which we cannot do justice to here. Nonetheless, a brief discussion of it is in order before concluding this section.

Not too many years ago it would have seemed self-evident that death occurs when circulation and respiration cease. As is well-known, medical technology (e.g., respirators) now has made it possible to maintain circulation and respiration long after other functions, such as sensory feeling, ability to think, motor control, consciousness, and so on, are irreversibly lost. Whether individuals who have lost these functions are still alive now is a difficult question to answer, a point for much discussion.

Why are we puzzled when we ask whether a client on a respirator, who no longer has sensory feeling, the ability to think, motor control, or consciousness, is still alive? No doubt many things, including what it means to die and what it is to be a living person. Reflection on our puzzlement will help us refine the issue. Fundamentally what we are asking is: Do we have a living person if the capacities for integrating the internal bodily environment and for integrating the self with the external environment through consciousness are irreversibly lost? (Cf. Veatch, 1976, pp. 21–54.) If we see them as the essential capacities, then an individual lacking these capacities is no longer a living person.

If this concept of death, or (what comes to the same thing) this concept of what it is to be a living person, is adopted, a new criterion for certifying death is necessary. Clearly, some clients will be dead despite the continuation of circulation and respiration. Others who lack the capacity to maintain circulation and respiration on their own will be alive with the aid of machines. If this is so, capacities other than circulation and respiration are the crucial ones, namely, the capacities for integrating the internal bodily environment and for integrating the self with the external environment through consciousness. These are capacities of the brain. Hence, the so-called "brain death" criterion has been offered as the test that best corresponds with the new understanding of death.

Since the brain is the seat of the capacities considered essential to human life, determination of its inability to carry out these functions indicates that death has occurred. One of several "brain death" criteria lists the following tests:

1. Unreceptivity and unresponsitivity
2. No movements or breathing

3. No reflexes
4. Flat electroencephalogram (Ad Hoc Committee, 1968, pp. 337–40)

The physician rather than the nurse has the grim task of declaring someone dead and thus of applying a criterion of death. But the nurse who has not thought carefully about the rationale for adopting a "brain death" criterion will be poorly prepared for effectively functioning in the final hours of a client's life. The fundamental issue that must be addressed by the nurse is philosophical: What is it to be a living human being? What are the essential features that must be present for a living being to be present?

The capacities for respiration and circulation are not the essential features. At most their absences are indicators that what is essential has been lost. The capacities for integration of the internal bodily environment and for integration of the self with the external environment through consciousness clearly are more essential and central to being a living human being. If so, our concept of death is simply the irreversible loss of these capacities. One who has suffered this irreversible loss is dead.

One of the great tragedies of modern life is that we are not always able to let the dead (as just defined) be given a decent and timely burial. Bodies remain attached to constantly monitored machines, while others argue about the legality of turning off the machines or the rights of health professionals or family members to do so. Some in positions of power or influence continue to insist that the body is not dead while blood and oxygen are still circulating. Those who recognize the presence of death find this behavior ghoulish and disrespectful of the person who once was.

It is not surprising that many find it difficult to accept that death has come if respiration and circulation can be mechanically induced. For years the heart-lung criterion was accepted without question. It is part of our way of thinking. I suspect another reason also plays a crucial role, namely, the fear of premature burial or of being treated as dead when one is not. This fear may blind many so that they fail to see the moral repugnance of erring on the other side by adopting too confining a criterion—one that allows those who are dead to be treated as if they were alive. What is required is to steer a steady middle course that avoids the Scylla of prematurely declaring a person dead and the Charybdos of treating a cadaver as if it were a living person.

The Nurse and the Aged and Chronically Ill Patient

In Chapter 2 we noted that people of advanced age and the chronically ill with diminished capacities are more likely than others to need the nurture, the care, the emotional support, the long-term monitoring, and the training that nurses are well-suited to provide. The ailing aged and the chronically ill need *care* and sustenance. As was pointed out earlier, for these clients, highly technical and interventionist skills of the physician are really ancillary to the caring function of the nurse.

In this chapter, we shall discuss some of the fundamental moral issues that arise in nursing care of the aged and chronically ill. The fundamental concern of respect for persons, of maintaining client autonomy, of course is also the key issue in the moral treatment of these clients. A separate issue that takes us beyond the perspective of the care-providing staff nurse is also raised: the question of justice in providing care for the elderly and chronically ill as opposed to those with acute illnesses. The issue of justice will be introduced here and discussed further in Chapter 8 (which deals with justice and health care delivery).

We begin with a recitation of facts about the changing median age of the population and its relation to nursing care. The number of persons sixty-five years of age or older has increased dramatically in this century. The growth in numbers has clearly out-paced the increase in the population at large, and this trend will continue, barring a catastrophic event or radical change in life-expectancy. As the persons born in the "baby boom" of the 1950s and 1960s reach old age, the number will again surge upward.

Many elderly have no need for special health care and remain physically and psychologically intact to the end of their lives. A vast number have no need to limit their major activities for reasons of health. The elderly as a group are done a disservice if we project on all of them the difficulties and limitations experienced by some. We must keep this in mind as we focus our attention on the minority of elderly persons who are in need of nursing care.

Some statistics and distinctions may help us maintain this perspective. Currently, approximately 20 to 22 million Americans are over the age of sixty-five. This is about 10 to 11 percent of the total population. At the turn of the century, only about 4 percent of the population were over sixty-five. Gerontologists find it useful to distinguish between the "young-old" and the "old-old"—between the retired persons in their late fifties, sixties, and early seventies who are relatively healthy and vigorous and seek meaningful ways to use their time, and those persons in their mid-seventies, eighties, and nineties who generally need a wide range of supportive and restorative health and social services. Of the "young-old"—the larger group—less than 25 percent need to limit their major activities for reasons of health. Of the "old-old," the majority have health problems that adversely affect their functioning. No more than 1.5 million of the 20 to 22 million over the age of sixty-five suffer from senility (i.e., show symptons of mental deterioration, such as loss of memory, loss of ability to do simple calculations, and disorientation of time and place) (Goldman, 1978). Clearly then, not all the elderly in institutions or under home care suffer from senility. The common stereotype of the elderly patient as senile is a faulty and dangerous generalization.

The following summarizes the situation well:

> The majority of older Americans below the age of seventy-five are independent. Among those not in this majority, and among those seventy-five years of age and older, intractable problems of ill health are prevalent, straining to the limit the resources of the health-care delivery system, and exposing its deficiencies. In the United States the sick aged (bedfast and housebound) number more than three million, or between twelve and fourteen percent of those over sixty-five. Elderly patients remain in hospital twice as long and require hospitalization twice as often as those under sixty-five. They account for one-fourth of the nation's health expenditures, are the prime users of long-term care facilities, and consume twenty-five percent of all drugs. Unfortunately, the emphasis in American society has been on "high medical technology" designed to meet acute, episodic needs, rather than on adequate care for the chronically ill. Yet, as one commentator observes, "While the aged have need for acute medical care, their major requirement is in the continuum of services for the chronically disabled that will enable them to function optimally" [Young, 1978, p. 65].

When we speak of the special problems of the elderly, it is convenient to speak in terms of age categories. Nevertheless, a person's chronological age does not have as much to do with his or her problems of aging as do the cellular, physical, and organic changes (thickening of the lenses of the eyes, increased problems with joints, thinning and graying of hair, auto-immunity problems, brittleness of bones, lack of agility, and so on) and the degree of psychological and mental changes (rigidity of thought, difficulty with memory and attention, inability to cope with new ideas and situations, "living in the past," and so on), all of which we associate with advanced age.

Given that many of the ailing elderly have these age-related traits as well as other medical problems, they often need special treatment and are particularly dependent. These factors—special needs and dependency—are the source of two of the most vexing moral issues related to care for the elderly, namely, the problem of the just distribution of health care resources and the problem of avoiding the infringement of autonomy of particularly vulnerable and dependent clients.

First we shall turn to the issue of the fair use of resources for the treatment of the chronically ill and ailing elderly. Currently (as we have seen) the elderly account for a disproportionate percentage of our nation's total health care expenditures—roughly 11 percent of the population, utilizing approximately 30 percent of the resources. Is this an appropriate use of limited resources? For example, should we give blood to an eighty-five-year-old who is on a death projection and is suffering from dementia (senility)? What about antibiotics? What about renal dialysis in case of kidney malfunction? What about resuscitative measures if he or she stops breathing?

In actual practice, where the aged or chronically ill client is makes a difference in how vigorously he or she is treated. The same client would likely be treated differently in a hospital than in a nursing home. Whether or not a policy is explicitly formulated, decisions concerning the level of treatment are made by health care professionals on the basis of the clients' ages, their life-prospects, their past, and their family relationships. Informal networks of physicians, nurses, social workers, and other professionals form, and a collective decision (perhaps not even explicitly stated) is made concerning the appropriate level of treatment in individual cases. For example, it may be decided not to treat a particular elderly person's fever after considering that she is bedridden, in pain, unmarried, and alone. A decision not to treat for these reasons would be made more readily in a nursing home than in a hospital. But in either type of facility such decisions are made.

If decisions concerning the treatment of the ailing elderly and chronically ill are being made on the bases of age, life-prospects, quality of life, and so on, we must ask whether these factors are *morally relevant* ones. That is, are these factors appropriate bases upon which to make decisions to treat or not to treat?

Consider the various issues that could be seen as relevant to treatment decisions concerning the ailing elderly or the chronically ill: (1) the client's wishes; (2) the client's best interests; (3) the wishes of the family; (4) the best interests of the family; (5) the client's life expectancy; (6) the prognosis of the disease; (7) the degree of disability that will remain (including mental and physical disabilities); (8) the chance of cure (can the treatment improve the client's condition or is it merely palliative?); (9) the presence of other problems and their prognoses (with the elderly it is especially common that there are several different problems rather than just one faulty system or infection); and (10) the cost of treatment.

Good reasons can be given for considering each of these ten factors. In fact, it may be that we are acting irresponsibly if we do not take all of them into account. Yet on the other hand, it may seem morally inappropriate to base a decision not to treat on such things as its cost or the best interests of the family (rather than solely on the client's).

To resolve this dilemma, it is useful to distinguish the therapeutic context (the health professional–client relationship), on the one hand, and the public policy context (the legislative and health facility administration), on the other. Some of these factors are properly considered on the one level and others are not, and vice versa.

As is well known, presently a large portion of our gross national product goes to health care. Obviously, the money spent for health care is not available for other needs, such as education, police protection, maintenance of roads and parks. As we have seen, the cost of treating the elderly is out of proportion to their numbers. A responsible social policy must recognize limits and balance diverse needs both within the health care budget and relative to other worthy expenditures. Each health care facility also has limited resources. Responsible administration will make allocation decisions concerning categories of clients—e.g., various accident victims and other acutely ill clients, chronically ill and aged clients. Factors such as the prognosis for cure and a return to a full life, the client's life expectancy, the cost of treatment, and the presence of other problems and complications must be taken into account in formulating treatment policy.

Surely it is not morally objectionable to make these kinds of calculations and base policy upon them. What is objectionable, however, is when bedside decisions are made on these bases. These are general policy decisions and are not to be made on an individual basis in the therapeutic context. The health professional's fundamental if not sole concern *qua* provider of care must be to do the best he or she can for each client—especially acting to maximize each client's autonomy. His or her practice, of course, must be carried out within the confines and limits of the general policies that have been adopted. For example, the health care team should not be deciding on an individual basis whether blood should be given to a senile eighty-five-year-old when it might better be used to help a twenty-four-year-old accident victim. If blood is in short supply, however, general policies should be in place to ensure the most efficient and fair use of resources.

The standard for these *policy* decisions will be discussed in a later chapter. In this chapter we shall focus on the therapeutic decision. As has been argued in other sections of the book, the client's own wishes clearly are a relevant factor in decisions concerning an individual's care. The position we have defended makes this a primary consideration—one which can be set aside only if clear evidence can be given that the client is incompetent or temporarily unable to articulate a position consistent with his or her own fundamental values. (This is an implication of the autonomy principle and is to be defended and developed systematically in the section below on paternalism.)

Another factor, of fundamental concern to health professionals, is consideration of the client's best interests. Without infringing on the client's autonomy and right to self-determinism and within the confines of general policy, those in charge of a client's care must take the actions that promote the client's best interests rather than those of his or her family, the hospital, or the state. (As we have seen earlier, however, if a conflict remains between the competent client's consistent wishes and the health professional's judgment of what is best for that client, the client's wishes must be given priority.)

As with all other clients, the fundamental moral concern is that their dignity and self-identity be maintained. Because the predominant form of health care in the United States is acute rather than chronic, treatment of the chronically ill and ailing elderly often is less than optimal. The care that is provided threatens their individuality and autonomy. One reason for this is that the priority placed on acute care results in less time for clients with chronic illness. Another reason is that the incentives encourage treatment modalities that do not necessarily benefit the elderly and chronically ill. A hospital and physicians can readily increase their incomes if they use high technology. But what these clients more frequently need is human care to help them overcome physical discomfort and personal interaction. These lacks in the care of the chronically ill and elderly are the source of some of the greatest challenges to their autonomy. The (ill-suited) care, or lack of care, contributes to their deterioration and their dependency upon others.

If the moral objective of care is to preserve and enhance client autonomy (as we have been arguing), care that produces dependency when it could be avoided must be criticized. Dependency undermines autonomy. Dependency can lead to humiliation. It can result in undue loss of dignity, of freedom, and the ability to make one's own choices. Moral considerations demand that, wherever possible, the elderly client be free to direct his or her own affairs. Given the prevalance of the stereotype of the elderly client as frail and possibly senile or at least "out of touch," well-meaning health professionals and the client's adult children usurp the responsibilities many of the elderly and chronically ill can still carry out. They make choices for the elderly which they are quite capable of making. Retaining as much responsibility as they can handle, especially in the care of themselves, on the other hand, enhances their autonomy and sense of self-worth.

The aging process itself (e.g., lack of agility, increased problems with joints, thickening of the lenses of the eyes), the age-related roles we are socialized into playing, the government-sponsored social services for the elderly, the structure and operating procedures of institutions (hospitals, nursing homes) that care for the elderly: *all* of these contribute to dependency. Unless those providing health care make a concerted effort to counteract these forces, an ailing elderly (and also a chronically ill) person is likely to be overwhelmed. He or she is simply compelled to accept a life of dependency, despite the concomitant indignity and humiliation.

Institutionalization will undermine elderly persons' autonomy if, in one way or another, it is communicated to them that, for example, their nurses—not they themselves—are now to make all decisions for them. If being in the nurses' care requires that they allow others to make their decisions for them, the ailing elderly or chronically ill person has no choice. He or she cannot continue without the nursing assistance. Accepting dependency no matter how humiliating seems better than being abandoned and without the help so desperately needed.

The nurses who step in and take charge may be doing this with the highest motives. Yet their action is morally remiss, for they are failing to respect the client as a person. As we argued in an earlier chapter, the morally proper role for the nurse is to help the client, wherever possible, to help himself or herself. The principle which must guide nurses' behavior is to exercise no more control over the client than is consistent with an objective assessment of the client's physical and mental limitations. Only in those areas in which it is clear that the client cannot act for himself or herself is the nurse free to act on his or her behalf. To know where the line is takes nursing skill and experience. Good intentions applied without nursing ability and discernment are not sufficient for the moral practice of nursing.

One of the bases for assuming that elderly clients are unable to act in their own best interest is the fact that their values are often quite different from those of younger persons. These different values arise from a perspective that is especially at variance with that of the younger health professional. "For example, it is often difficult to persuade an elderly, critically ill nursing home patient to go to the hospital, leaving a known protective environment of peers, nurses, the familiar begonia on a radiator sill, a favorite aid, and the reliable routine of a final lifestyle—in short, home" (Ratzan, 1980, p. 34).

The feeling of security and belonging may be far more important to the elderly person than the possibility of staving off death for a few extra months or even years. Whereas many younger persons fear (premature) death and will go to great lengths in their struggle against it, many an elderly person (especially one who has lived a full life) does not share this fear but fears much more the possibility of a lingering, lonely, agonizing, or depersonalized death.

In *The Dilemmas of Care: Social and Nursing Adaptions to the Deformed, the Disabled and the Aged,* R. P. Preston describes the very sick and elderly client as follows: "He grieves for his entire generation and likely sees scant temporal prospects for himself. He cannot do anything as he once did. He is dependent with minimal opportunity to serve. Life sputters and horizons narrow to immediate comforts and discomforts" (Preston, 1979, p. 154). We have emphasized the importance of preserving as much of the elderly client's freedom and autonomy as possible. Equally important, if we are to respect them as persons, is protecting their identity—an identity derived from the past. As Preston states, these clients see "scant temporal prospects" for themselves. If anything can, their past will help them find meaning and satisfaction.

In contrast, younger persons are far more likely to find meaning and make decisions in terms of the future. The early years of one's life are all geared to the future. From nursery school to college and career training, one is preparing for the future. The decisions of those beginning careers and families are all made with an eye toward the future. Sacrifices are made for the future. For many people, and especially for the ambitious professional, the future is the focal point of nearly all one's activities. The situation is quite different for the ailing elderly client. Awareness of these different perspectives is necessary if a younger person is going to respect the elderly as persons. For someone eager to move on to the future, the tendency of the elderly to retell stories about persons and events from the past can be exasperating and seem a waste of time. Yet, for the elderly client who is likely to be socially isolated and may even be one of the last survivors of his or her generation and circle of friends, retelling stories from the past puts him or her in contact with what has meaning and value. If these memories are not preserved, the self is lost. By sharing these memories (i.e., by listening) the health professional can make contact with the client as a person.

Since elderly persons' senses of self are tied to the past, one way to assist them in maintaining their integrity (their identity) is to encourage them to retain personal belongings and momentos that remind them of persons and events of the past. In the following case, the nurse is very much aware of the need to protect the elderly client's identity and, with sensitivity and ingenuity, makes an important contribution to the care of her client:

Mrs. C. was an obese 92-year-old woman who was brought to the hospital from a nursing home. Her medical diagnosis was congestive heart failure, pulmonary edema and uncontrolled diabetes. She was admitted to Room 530 on my weekend off. When I arrived on the floor on Monday night she had been in the hospital for two days. As I was talking with the evening nurse, Mrs. C.

began calling, "Nurse, please. Nurse, please, Nurse, please." The evening nurse told me she called out like this all the time. She had been put into a private room "so we could close the door and she would not disturb the other patients."

I went to Room 530 to introduce myself to Mrs. C. and to tell her that if she needed anything to press the call button and I would come. Mrs. C. was fighting to get out of her restraints, had pulled off her oxygen mask, and was trying to climb over the siderails. I told her she had to stay in bed. "Your doctor ordered strict bed rest."

"But you don't understand," she said, "I have to go to my room."

"This is your room," I answered. "You're in the hospital now and this is your room."

"No, this isn't my room. I have to go to my room."

Mrs. C., who was alert and oriented during the day, became very confused and disoriented at night. I looked around the room to find something that belonged to her, something of hers that she could hold onto, something personal. But there was nothing. Her family had taken everything home.

I stayed with Mrs. C. and held her hand. She calmed down and slept for awhile. Often during the night she called, "Nurse, please. Nurse, please. Nurse, please." I would answer her immediately and she would say, "What are you doing here? I didn't call." She wet her bed twice during that night and when I changed her hospital gown, she didn't want me to put her soiled gown in the hamper. "I'll need it later," she said. She seemed to be comforted when I put the gowns in the closet. The closet was no longer empty.

When I gave report to the day staff that morning, I asked the day nurse if she ever saw any member of Mrs. C's. family. She said that Mrs. C's. daughter visited her every day and that she did have other visitors. I explained to the nurse what had happened during the night, and begged her to ask Mrs. C's. daughter to bring some personal belongings of her mother to the hospital. It would be of great comfort to Mrs. C.

Nothing was brought in. I left notes for the daughter. Nothing was done.

Mrs. C's. emotional and physical health deterioriated. Her anxiety kept her awake most of the night; and because of her medical problems, the doctor was reluctant to give her barbiturates. She became more dependent and less willing or able to help herself. She called out all night, "Nurse, please. Nurse, please. Nurse, please." There were times I wanted to scream at her to shut up! Of course, she couldn't understand that she was only one of eighteen patients, and that many of the other patients were complaining about the noise she made.

I began working days on a Sunday, two weeks after Mrs. C. was admitted. She was more lucid during the day and knew she was in the hospital. But by this time she would not even attempt to assist with her own care. If she weren't fed, she wouldn't eat. She was extremely depressed.

I waited for Mrs. C's. daughter that Sunday. I explained to her that her mother, like many older people, sometimes became confused at night, especially when placed in a new and stressful environment like the hospital. She needed something of her own to keep with her. The daughter understood immediately. She went home and brought her mother a shopping bag. In the bag was Mrs. C's. purse, her sweater, and a nightgown. She also brought a picture of the grandchildren. Mrs. C. held onto that bag all day. She slept with the shopping bag in her bed.

Each time a member of the family came to visit, he or she brought something for Mrs. C. The change in Mrs. C. was gradual. She seemed to regain her sense of self, to become aware of who and why she was. She even began feeding herself. [This very moving case was written by Ms. Andrea Cohen, a nurse and student of mine.]

The care provided in the previous case—care that exhibited both moral sensitivity and nursing skill—is in sharp contrast to that of the following:

One day while working on a large medical unit, I was attracted by a screaming protest: "Aeee! No! No! No! No!" I followed the noise to a patient's room wherein a husky nurse was force-feeding an old lady who was tied to a chair. The nurse mimed the patient's expressions and gestures, laughing as she did so. "Come on, Mamma, you haven't eaten all day." The patient screamed and the nurse scooted a spoonful of food into her mouth. The medication nurse came in behind me; we both surveyed the scene. The attending nurse warned, "Look out, you must stay out of range. She will spit her food out at you." The medication nurse circumspectly popped a pill into the patient's mouth and then added, "She's looking for someplace to spit that pill out—there." The pill and the food splattered on the floor. "I can't stand patients like that. She knows what she's doing." The two nurses continued to discuss the doctors' orders concerning the patient. Occasionally, the attending nurse cast a loud aside to the patient, accompanied by exaggerated gestures, "How's it going, Mamma?" [Preston, 1979, p. 175].

The fundamental difference between these two cases is the obvious respect for the client as a person in the former and the clear lack of regard for the client's feelings, rights, integrity, and autonomy in the latter. The nurses in the latter case have simply made a presumption that the client is senile. "As senility is a common malady of elderly patients, many nurses presume at the slightest sign of feebleness that an elderly person is feebleminded. Unless an elderly patient strongly demonstrates a normative mentality, license will likely be taken" (Preston, 1979, p. 175).

Perhaps there is no better reminder that the ailing elderly client is a person than the following note written by one. When this woman died in the geriatric ward of Ashludie Hospital near Dundee, Ireland, the nurse sorting her meager possessions found this poem:

> What do you see, nurses, what do you see?
> Are you thinking when you are looking at me:
> A crabbit old woman, not very wise,

Uncertain of habit, with far-away eyes.
Who dribbles her food and makes no reply
When you say in a loud voice, "I do wish you'd try."
Who seems not to notice the things that you do.
And forever is losing a stocking or shoe.
Who unresisting or not, lets you do as you will,
With bathing and feeding, the long day to fill.
Is that what you are thinking? Is that what you see?
Then open your eyes, nurse, you're not looking at me.
I'll tell you who I am as I sit here so still;
As I use at your bidding, as I eat at your will.
I'm a small child of ten with a father and mother,
Brothers and sisters, who love one another.
A young girl of sixteen with wings on her feet,
Dreaming that now soon a lover she'll meet.
A bride soon at twenty—my heart gives a leap,
Remembering the vows that I promised to keep;
At twenty-five now I have young of my own,
Who need me to build a secure, happy home;
A woman of thirty, my young now grow fast,
Bound to each other with ties that should last;
At forty my young sons have grown and are gone,
But my man's beside me to see I don't mourn.
At fifty, once more babies play round my knee.
Again we know children, my loved one and me.
Dark days are upon me, my husband is dead,
I look at the future, I shudder with dread,
For my young are all rearing young of their own,
And I think of the years and the love that I've known.
I'm an old woman now and nature is cruel—
'Tis her jest to make old age look like a fool.
The body it crumbles, grace and vigour depart,
There is now a stone where I once had a heart;
But inside this old carcass a young girl still dwells,
And now and again my battered heart swells.
I remember the joys, I remember the pain,
And I'm loving and living life over again.
I think of the years all too few—gone too fast.
And accept the stark fact that nothing can last.
So open your eyes, nurses, open and see
Not a crabbit old woman, look closer—see ME!*

Some elderly persons, reflecting on the life that was—remembering,
as does this woman, the joys of childhood and the responsibilities of

*I have not seen this poem in print. Copies were duplicated and distributed to the nurses
at the Ashludie Hospital. One of these copies, or more likely a copy of one of these
copies, was given to me.

young adulthood—find that the prospect of continued decline and possibly pain and isolation resulting from immobility and loss of communication skills is just too bleak to endure. Suicide is contemplated. Seneca (Roman statesman and philosopher, 4 BC–65 AD) stated well the position of the elderly person who sees suicide as the better course.

I will not relinquish old age if it leaves my better part intact. But if it begins to shake my mind, if it destroys my faculties one by one, if it leaves me not life but breath, I will depart from the putrid or the tottering edifice. If I know that I must suffer without hope of relief I will depart not through fear of the pain itself but because it prevents all for which I live [*De Ira*, i.15].

The increasing numbers of suicides among the elderly add this concern to all the others the nurse caring for elderly clients must consider. The question of suicide is especially difficult to address when the person contemplating suicide is elderly or chronically ill. To follow our natural and admirable inclination to prevent another human being from suicide may be the (morally) wrong thing to do with many of these clients.

Suppose that a nurse knows that an elderly client being discharged is likely to commit suicide for reasons such as Seneca expresses in the above quotation. Should the nurse take steps to prevent it—e. g., hold up the discharge so that the client can be kept under observation and treated by a psychiatrist? Or, out of respect for the client's freedom to choose his or her own destiny, should she refrain from intervention?

As is well documented, suicide attempts are frequently calls for help rather than straight-forward attempts to end one's life. Many times the suicide attempt is a high-risk game. Clearly, if one is desperately crying out for help, all things being equal, we should try to help. To grant the suicide attempter the right to end his or her life—when his or her aim is to make a dramatic play for help and not to die—is insensitive. To say that we must not intervene because it would violate his or her rights is a perversion of the autonomy principle.

With certain elderly clients, however, and this includes those who agree with Seneca, it is quite clear that they are not attempting suicide as a desperate means of getting help. Rather they do wish to die. They have thought long and hard about what they value and what is essential for life that is to be worth living. Their own prospects are extremely limited: they have lived their lives; many of those nearest to them have already died; they have discharged their responsibilities to their children. Continued existence offers little that is fulfilling while it could bring much that is painful and, even worse, degrading.

Suicide committed under circumstances such as these—resulting from deliberate choice after years of reflection—is called *rational suicide.* This is to be contrasted with suicide as a cry for help or as a sympton of depression resulting from a temporary setback.

In many actual cases it may not be clear how a likely suicide should be categorized. Is it a cry for help despite the appearance of deliberation over time and a reasonable desire to end it all? Or is it rational suicide? Professional expertise and experience with suicide attempters as well as an understanding of the particular client contribute to making this clinical judgment.

Of course, the proper moral response will be different depending on this clinical decision. A cry for help is answered, wherever possible, with a helping hand—which, in the case of a suicide attempt, involves preventing the client from acting as he or she intends. (For further discussion of this issue, see the discussion of paternalism, Chapter 5, part 2, below.) On the other hand, rational suicide requires a different response.

Intervention that restrains the client committing rational suicide cannot be defended, for it fails to respect autonomy. In keeping with respect for the client's right of self-determination, however, the nurse could question the client to make certain that he or she had considered all the possibilities, had accurately determined the probabilities, and so on. The nurse might express her or his own opinions and even dismay. Doing so is emphatically treating the client as a rational person. Such interaction meets the other as one who is able to think for himself or herself and is an indication that this ability is recognized and honored. But if the nurse goes beyond this and exercises his or her authority or power to prevent the discharge of the client or in other ways thwarts the client's ability to act, these are unwarranted acts of interference (despite their honorable motives). Included in this category would be attempts to revive the client should he or she be brought in after the attempt had been made and if it is evident that the client would die if left alone. Especially for persons strongly committed to saving lives and lengthening life-spans, this would not be an easy thing to do.

As people live longer and a greater percentage of our population is aged, an ever increasing proportion of nursing time will be spent caring for the elderly. The moral problems we have discussed in this chapter will be with us for many years to come. Much more must be done to prepare nurses for optimal service to this rapidly growing population.

5

Moral Restraints

From the basic principles of autonomy and respect for persons outlined in Chapter 1 flow several specific principles that form the core of a health professional ethics. In this chapter we shall examine four of these: the moral requirement of informed consent; the moral prohibition against paternalism; the moral duty to tell the truth; and the moral obligation to maintain client confidentiality. A philosophical discussion of the everyday moral issues of consent, coercion, candor, and confidentiality confronting nurses must justify and clarify the principles upon which decisions are to be made. We shall show how principles offering moral guidance on these issues can be derived from the basic moral position that has been defended in Chapter 1. And, having done that, we shall discuss how these principles are to be applied in actual cases. We begin with consent.

Is Informed Consent Always Morally Required?

Often, legal and moral requirements do not coincide. With regard to informed consent, however, we are in the happy position of having the law require what morality also requires. Concerning the requirement of informed consent, both law and morality (as developed here) appeal to the same basic principle, self-determination. Medical intervention on competent adults legally and morally requires their voluntary and informed consent. In the words of Judge Spotswood W. Robinson, II, in *Canterbury v. Spence:* "The root premise is the concept, fundamental in American jurisprudence, that '[e]very human being of adult years and sound mind has a right to determine what shall be done with his own body' " (Robinson, 1972, p. 79). Justice Alfred Schroeder of the Kansas Supreme Court also expressed the legal standards for informed consent by appealing to the basic principle of self-determinism:

Anglo-American law starts with the premise of thorough-going self-determination. It follows that each man is considered to be master of his own body, and he may, if he be of sound mind, expressly prohibit the performance of life-saving surgery, or other medical treatment. A doctor might well believe that an operation or form of treatment is desirable or necessary but the law does not permit him to substitute his own judgment for that of the patient by any form of artifice or deception [Veatch, 1976, p. 117].

Although the specific legal requirements vary from state to state, the basic requirements are clear and constant.

In medical practice through the ages it has been recognized that a person's consent is necessary to his or her being a patient (client). "It is the patient's prerogative to accept medical treatment or take his chances of living without it" (Plant, 1968, p. 650). A consequence of this (and one that is often difficult to accept) is that withdrawal of that consent terminates his or her being a client.

Since the right of a competent adult client to refuse or discontinue treatment is firmly established, challenges to a client's wishes not to be treated usually are based on the question of competency. If the client is incompetent (a notion to be clarified later), one is not violating the requirement of informed consent in subverting his or her wishes. Informed consent is not possible for an incompetent client and, therefore, one cannot be required to obtain it.

Deciding whether a client is incompetent is very difficult. This difficulty makes it possible to use the competency issue as a way of circumventing the requirement of informed consent. In some cases a client is placed in a catch-22 dilemma. If he or she does not acquiesce in the physician's judgment and rejects treatment, this is taken to be sufficient ground for being judged incompetent. If, to be judged competent, the client must acquiese, then being competent is of little value. There are situations in which rejection of treatment would be utterly unreasonable. But surely the mere fact that a person rejects treatment (even lifesaving treatment) is not enough to establish incompetence.

Before we see how the requirement of informed consent can be clarified and applied to actual situations, let us see how it is grounded in the fundamental moral principle of respect for individuals as autonomous beings capable of making decisions and acting on them.

In Chapter 1 we argued that the fundamental basis of morality is the fact that human beings have dignity and worth that is unique. We saw that as such human beings are never to be used merely as means but always at the same time as ends.

The duty of obtaining informed consent before engaging in medical treatment or initiating any invasive procedures follows from the duty to respect persons as rational beings and as ends, not merely as means. If we fail to acquaint the client with what is going on, we treat him or her as less than a human being. Although motivated by a desire to help, our action toward the competent client we keep uninformed is manipulative and evidence of a lack of awareness of the client as a rational being.

Some years ago when I was going "on rounds" in a teaching hospital, we would examine a client, stop at the foot of the bed, quietly discuss his or her case, and then without offering any real explanation to the client move on to the next case. I became painfully aware of the ease with which basic moral demands of respect for persons can be overlooked by well-meaning, overworked health professionals. Surely failure to inform these clients of what is going on exhibits a lack of regard for them as persons, no matter how desirous the health professionals are to cure the disease. Recognition of clients as persons entails recognition of their capacities for rational decision-making and for action consequent upon their decision.

In many respects it is far worse when one's humanity is ignored than when one is treated unfairly or unkindly. In the latter case, at least one's existence has been acknowledged and one has been given a basis for asserting oneself. It is far more likely that health professionals will simply fail to recognize that the client is a person with feelings, fears, aspirations, and hopes like their own than that they will be rude and insulting. Were they insulting, the client could simply and angrily dismiss them. The anger might even be therapeutic. But when the health professional treats a client as a nonentity, or as an object, or as merely a diseased body, she or he has struck a powerful blow at the client's identity. Failure to provide information to the client about his or her condition is one of the most effective ways of striking this blow, whatever one's intent.

Obviously a client must have information about his or her condition in order to exercise rational choice. Beside being too busy and preoccupied to provide information, another reason that health professionals sometimes withhold information is the desire to make the decision for the person, feeling that their own decision will be better. To do that is inconsistent with the principle of autonomy, for the competent client is the one to decide. From a moral point of view, his or her uncoerced informed choice is essential. As Paul Ramsey says, "No man is good enough to cure another without his consent" (Ramsey, 1970, p. 7). We do not have the moral right to impose on another our views of that person's happiness or of how that person can best live his or her life.

Usually it is the physician who is legally required to see to it that the client has given consent for a proposed treatment. In the practice of numerous physicians and institutions, as nurses frequently report, the consent obtained is neither informed nor truly voluntary. The nurse is left to answer the client's many questions after a doctor has hurriedly obtained consent. It may even be evident to the nurse that, although the client signed a consent form, he or she has no clear understanding of the procedure. In some institutions, in contrast, the nurse is given the task of obtaining the signature on the consent form. Whatever the particular circumstances, the nurse is involved in the process of obtaining consent. Hence, in order to perform his or her job well, the nurse must have a clear understanding of the legal and moral require-ments of informed consent. Here we shall focus on the moral require-ments.

The requirements of informed consent are best understood by an examination of its three key elements: (1) When is consent *informed* consent, and how much information is needed? (2) When is consent fully *voluntary* consent? (3) Who is *competent* to give consent?

The following three cases exemplify these three basic elements: (1) Consider the case of a client suffering from breast cancer. She agrees to have a radical mastectomy but is not told that studies indicate that it may be no more effective than much less radical surgery. Has she been given adequate information to have made an informed choice? (2) A client's physician says that immediate surgery would be the best course of action and that other possible alternatives really are not worth considering. Given the physician's position of authority and power, is the client able to make a truly voluntary or uncoerced decision? (3) A client is in great pain, is bedridden, is suffering from cancer, and is fearful that he is a burden to his family. Is such a person functioning normally enough to be considered a rational decision-maker, one who is able to determine what is best for himself?

Anyone who has worked as a nurse or other health professional knows how difficult it is to meet the requirements of informed consent. There are many times when a nurse is bound to feel that the requirement (especially as we shall develop it here) is too rigorous. Most clients will lack education, will fail to grasp information pro-vided, or will be emotionally unstable. To obtain "full" informed consent will be an unattainable ideal. Still, by requiring that nothing can be done to them without their informed consent, we recognize their humanity and respect their autonomy. We acknowledge that they are persons with their own interests, not objects to be manipulated either to serve their own good or anyone else's.

Now let's turn to a more complete discussion of these elements, beginning with the information component. Since this is the aspect of informed consent that most involves the nurse, the greatest amount of time will be spent on it. The issue has already been before us. The Jolene Tuma case which we discussed in the introduction is a vivid example of a nurse's unavoidable involvement in the issue of the proper presentation of information to the client. In addition to discussion of the Tuma case, we shall examine three cases in which nurses are confronted with the question of whether adequate information has been given to the client.

(A)

A patient was admitted to the hospital for diagnostic procedures for a chest ailment. He had been suffering chest pains, shortness of breath and increasing fatigue for some time. Many tests were performed and the patient was given medications and treatment for emphysema. However, the physician had not discussed the diagnosis, treatment or prognosis with the patient.

The patient kept asking the staff nurse for information. She felt reluctant to discuss the matter with the patient until the physician had at least outlined the essential items. The nurse normally expected to help the patient learn about this illness but not until after the physician had disclosed the diagnosis.

As the days continued the physician did not respond precisely to the patient's questions. Neither did the physician respond to the nurse's suggestions that the patient be informed.

One day when the patient refused the medications and treatments, the nurse told the patient his diagnosis. She then proceeded to discuss the prognosis if the treatment regimen was followed carefully and the prognosis if he did not continue the treatment as ordered.

The patient again was cooperative with the nurse when she treated him. However, the physician severely reprimanded the nurse for her forwardness in assuming what, he said, was the physician's rightful role. He felt the patient should not have known his diagnosis or his prognosis. The nurse felt she was justified in telling him. He had a right to know. His care required his cooperation if he was to have any relief [Tate, 1977, pp. 27–28].

In this first case, virtually no information was given for days, and then it was given only because the lack of it had produced an untenable situation.

In the next case, some crucial information is withheld, information about possible alternatives and possible adverse side effects of the chosen alternative.

(B)

A 15-year-old patient was admitted for a total abdominal hysterectomy. She was an educable, mentally handicapped student with an IQ of 62. While preparing the patient for surgery which was to be done the next day, I talked with her mother. I was informed that the patient often exhibited undesirable suggestive sexual behavior when around persons of the opposite sex. She also neglected personal hygiene during her menstrual period but there was no history of menstrual problems.

In talking with the doctor, I learned that the patient's mother had requested the hysterectomy. She had stated that she did not have time and patience to teach the "slow" daughter how to take care of personal needs during her monthly periods. The patient's mother had stated that she felt it would be easier for the daughter to have a hysterectomy.

I explained to the mother the hormonal functions of the uterus and ovaries, that the patient could have problems resulting from the removal of them, and that an IQ of 62 was not too low to learn many things with adequate understanding and help. I also explained that a tubal ligation would produce sterility without the danger of hormonal problems later.

The patient's mother stated that she did not fully understand what was done in the two procedures but had requested the hysterectomy to which the surgeon had agreed. Before the operative permit was signed, the doctor was called. With much reluctance, the procedure order was changed to a tubal ligation. The doctor had not adequately informed the patient and her mother. This would have been unnecessary surgery [Carroll and Humphrey, 1979, pp. 168–169].

In the next case we see a common, but seldom defensible, reason being offered for failing to provide information, in this case to the parents of a child: that the client's representative lacks the requisite intelligence.

(C)

Mr. S and his wife have been visiting their 10-year-old daughter, Tina, daily since she was admitted to the hospital four days ago. She has a diagnosis of cancer of the liver, but the parents who are on welfare have not been told the diagnosis. The physician feels that the parents, who are Spanish speaking, will not comprehend any of the terminology necessary to understand the diagnosis. The nurses on the unit have described the parents as "dull," but feel that they should have an explanation of Tina's illness in order to give the required informed consent for various procedures. Both Mr. and Mrs. S have asked the nurses about what is going to happen to Tina. They know that Tina is critically ill [Aroskar and Davis, 1978, p. 207].

I suspect that, in these three cases, the reader will agree with the involved nurses that the information provided to the client is not adequate. We have seen that providing information is a moral requirement, for it is the way we show respect for the personhood and the self-determination of the client. Information must be provided so that the client can make an intelligent or rational decision. Enough information has been given only if the information provided puts the client in such a position.

Generally speaking, to be in such a position the client or responsible proxy would want to be informed about:

1. the procedures to be followed if the proposed course of treatment is pursued;

2. the likely results of the proposed treatment;

3. the attendant discomforts and risks as well as the expected benefits of the proposed treatment;

4. the possible alternatives to the proposed treatment along with a report of their risks and benefits; and

5. the likely results if the client remains untreated.

In some cases it may not be possible to provide answers to all these questions. For example, the outcome of the procedure may be unpredictable. If so, the client must be told just that. Lacking the information, which only the health professionals (and in some cases specifically the doctor) can provide, the client cannot make an informed decision. The health professional, and not the typical client, is trained to judge the hoped-for benefits from a proposed treatment, what risks are entailed, and what is the probability of success. For the client to make an intelligent choice, the health professional must share her or his professional expertise.

One of the common features of the three examples cited is the reluctance on the part of the physicians to do this. (Of course, not all physicians are reluctant to share their knowledge with their clients. Such cases are not discussed here because they are far less likely to raise moral problems for the nurse.) The physicians in the cases cited would probably agree with Franz Ingelfinger that "the trouble with informed consent is that it is not educated consent [and] the chances are remote that the subject really understands what he has consented to" (Ingelfinger, 1972, p. 465). Given their lack of confidence that the client can really understand explanations of procedures and alternatives, they do not make an effort to provide the full information we have argued is essential for the client to make a choice based on reason. In the interests of proceeding with the treatment program which, in their judgment, is best for the client, they do not want to risk having the client make a choice in favor of a less-desirable alternative.

In the three examples, the nurses have good evidence to support their beliefs that adequate information has not been offered. In each case the requirements we have outlined have been violated. In case A, the client has been given no reason to accept the rigors of the treatment. None of the information listed above, which is an essential foundation for a rational choice, has been provided. Not only has this client's autonomy and right to self-determination been violated, the lack of information has resulted in inadequate health care. Clearly, a client advocate would take steps to rectify the situation, as, in fact, the nurses did.

Case B raises a number of vexing questions. One of these, the right to give proxy consent, will be set aside while we focus on the requirements to discuss possible side-effects and available alternative forms of treatment. Not knowing about these (given the values and perspective of the mother), the hysterectomy appears to her to be the best course. But in this case, the additional information makes evident that the tubal ligation is the preferred option. Had the physician felt the moral demand to discuss the possible side-effects and to explore alternatives with the client's mother, she might also have come to realize that there was a better alternative than the one initially selected. Not only do the requirements of full information protect the client's autonomy; they also go some way toward improving health care.

Surely there are numerous clients and families of clients who are unable to comprehend even the most elementary explanation of a disease and the proposed treatment plan. Nevertheless, as in a court of law in which one's innocence is presumed until proven otherwise, the client's ability to comprehend and understand what is going on and to be able to make a judgment based on the data must be presumed until firm evidence establishes the contrary. In case C, the language and cultural barriers—which admittedly make communication more difficult—are excuses for ignoring the moral obligation to provide the information necessary for client choice. Is it really impossible to find someone conversant in Spanish and knowledgeable about medicine who can discuss with them in nontechnical terms Tina's diagnosis and prospects? Only then can they make rational choices concerning treatment decisions as well as sensible determinations on other family matters.

We began the book with a discussion of a case in which a nurse's acting on her belief that the client had not given truly informed consent resulted in her being dismissed from her job. She believed that the possible alternative treatments, including ones that she herself could not recommend, should be discussed with the client. In their fear that having this information would result in the client choosing a course of action other than the one they thought preferable, the physician and the client's family argued that the nurse overstepped her authority when, without recommending any particular course of action, she responded to questions about alternative forms of treatment, including unorthodox therapies such as laetrile, herb, nutrition, and touch therapies. Certainly, if we see the nurse as a client advocate, we must challenge their narrow conception of the nurse's role. That question has already been discussed, however, and is not the central issue in this chapter. Instead, the issue is what information the client is entitled to have as a basis upon which to decide whether to follow treatment plan x, y, or z—or perhaps none at all. We have argued that the client is entitled to whatever information is necessary for making an intelligent decision. Even if we are convinced that particular alternatives are not advisable or even are dangerous, if, as in this case, the client inquires about them, we must be prepared to discuss their merits and demerits. This does not mean that a health professional must give a client encouragement if he or she is intent upon a dangerous or foolish course of action. As long as the information is provided in as straightforward a way as possible, it would not be a violation of the client's autonomy to indicate—and give one's reasons for—one's own opinion as to which alternative is preferable and to warn against the dangers or folly of other alternatives. Willingness to state one's viewpoint while providing reasons for it can be a supreme expression of the respect one has for the autonomy and assertiveness of the other. Properly done, stating one's position is not coercive, nor need it be a subtle way of imposing one's own will upon another.

Yet there is always the danger that it will have an inhibiting, rather than an enhancing effect. How can one guard against violating the client's autonomy in this way? The most important thing to keep in mind is a distinction between the scientific or strictly medical judgments a health professional makes, on the one hand, and his or her value and life-style judgments, on the other. For example, it may be clear from the available data on success rates of various treatment modalities that surgery is the recommended treatment from the point of view of life-expectancy. Whether the resulting disfigurement the surgery entails is too heavy a burden to bear in exchange for the extra months or years gained is a question of a different order. This must be answered from the perspective of the client's values and interests. One's scientific knowledge, including an examination of recent research results, does not provide a basis for answering the latter question (although it does the former). In attempting to make such a value decision for a client, one is not exercising one's medical expertise; one is trying to make a life-style decision for another. In usurping the client's prerogative, not only is one overstepping his or her professional expertise, but one is also violating the client's right to self-determination. But if the health professional works with the client and helps him or her to see the choices within the framework of his or her (the client's) own values and disvalues (in some cases it may be necessary to help the client determine what these are) and on this ground recommends a course of action, the nurse or other health professional has helped the client exercise autonomy.

We have seen what conditions must be satisfied if a client is to have adequate information in order to make a rational decision concerning his or her health care. We have also seen how the manner in which the information is presented can restrain or enhance the possibility of a client's free choice or consent. Now we shall focus on the consent side of the informed consent requirement. In addition to the information we have said is morally required, what else is necessary to insure that the consent is truly voluntary? Clearly, one could have all the information we have said must be provided and still not be in a position to make a free choice, to act on one's own volition. For example, suppose a client is informed of all the possible alternatives but then, rather than being given a choice, is simply told that she must sign the form before her. The doctors are going to begin treatment Plan Y at once.

Some have argued that any client who is incapacitated, hospitalized due to illness, and under duress is in no position to act voluntarily. The strangeness and uncertainty of the situation are said to make a free choice impossible. For example, Ingelfinger (who was quoted earlier) says, "Incapacitated and hospitalized because of illness, frightened by strange and impersonal routines, and fearful for his health and perhaps life, he is far from exercising a free power of choice when the person on whom he anchors all his hopes [proposes a particular procedure]" (Ingelfinger, 1972, p. 466). He concludes that the process of obtaining informed consent in a hospital setting is "no more than an elaborate ritual."

This challenge must be taken seriously. There is no question that clients are often cowed by the authority of health professionals and the awesomeness of the modern, technically sophisticated hospital. Certainly these factors predispose a client's meek acquiescence to any order, suggestion, or request made by a member of the health care team. Who can stand up to such overwhelming forces?

The only hope for most clients to exercise their volition in this setting is to have allies within the institution, namely, professionals who want to help them to affirm their own values and to determine their own destinies. Instead of concluding (with physicians such as Ingelfinger) that the factors mentioned above defeat the ideal of informed consent, what is required is greater commitment and effort to realize it. The charge to the nurse to act as client advocate could not be made more clearly or more urgently. The moral importance of the nurse's role as we have developed it is evident.

Consider the following two rather blatant examples of the misuse of professional and institutional power to the detriment of the client's right to consent or dissent.

(D)

One morning while receiving the report from the third shift nurse, it was learned that a new admission to the hospital was scheduled for an angiogram. At that time, angiograms were not done at this hospital and patients were taken to a hospital in another town approximately 25 miles away from this service.

Everything seemed normal until the nurse on duty saw the patient, Mrs. B., who was a large woman weighing well over 200 pounds and who was very disturbed. The night nurse had tried to explain the procedure to her, but in her mental state she did not or could not comprehend. The nurses did not know if she was disturbed about having the angiogram or if she was disturbed for other reasons, but she was objecting very loudly to the procedure. . . .

Ms. B. would not listen to anyone. It was impossible to explain the need for the angiogram. When the physician was told that Mrs. B. was refusing the procedure, he went to see the patient, and then hastily said, "Aw, hell, we'll just snow her and take her on." One of the two nurses present told the doctor that this should not be done [Carroll and Humphrey, 1979, pp. 34–35].

(E)

Mrs. R is a woman in her mid-forties with multiple sclerosis. She has two teen-age daughters, fourteen and sixteen years old, living at home. Mr. R, a middle-management executive in a local firm, left the home five years ago. Mrs. R often comes into the emergency room of the local community hospital for treatment of acute episodes of asthma. The physician has ordered that if Mrs. R arrests during an acute episode, no CODE should be called. As far as the nurses know, the physician made this decision on his own with no input from the patient or others significant to her or depending on her. One nurse is terribly upset because this decision conflicts strongly with her own professional and personal moral values. She herself has said on several occasions that Mrs. R's home situation is "intolerable" and "I certainly wouldn't want to live under those circumstances." None of the nurses have heard Mrs. R express any similar feelings about her situation even though she usually seems somewhat depressed when she comes into the emergency room [Aroskar and Davis, 1978, pp. 207–8].

Although there are many borderline cases in which it is extremely difficult, if not impossible, to determine whether a person is acting freely, these are not such cases. Here there can be no doubt that the client is not free. Yet neither these people's illnesses nor the institution itself need inevitably lead to situations such as these. Blatant disregard for a client's right to consent or dissent is not a necessary outcome of illness or institutionalization.

In case D, the physician could have waited to proceed with the diagnostic test in the hopes that the client would become calmer later and the procedure could be explained and comprehended—at which point the client could decide. On the other hand, if she remained in an agitated state and was judged incompetent, appropriate steps could be taken, as we shall discuss shortly.

The case of the woman with multiple sclerosis is all too representative of decision-making concerning clients whose life-prospects are bleak. Again, nothing in the setting or the condition of the client makes it impossible to discuss the situation with her and to let *her* decide whether or not she would want resuscitative measures initiated should she suffer cardiac arrest during an acute episode of asthma.

Sometimes, if we are in a philosophical mood, we may wonder if any of our actions are really free. We have probably all had experiences in which actions that seemed free at the time later appeared not to have been free at all. It is logically possible that free will (autonomous choice) is an illusion. Yet none of us really lives that way. We agonize over choices. We feel that our deliberation really makes a difference and that, often, we could have acted differently than we did. We can feel the difference between times when our choice is the determining factor and when someone else's is. We resent others imposing their wills upon us because we believe they could do otherwise; they are not compelled to interfere.

Many times, especially when serious illness strikes, we see that—if we are to act rationally—we really have but one alternative, e.g., only one alternative offers any real promise, or only one alternative is even acceptable. In a sense, then, we have no choice in the matter. For example, with a ruptured appendix we may have no rational choice other than surgery. But even in situations of no choice, we can and do distinguish between those in which impersonal forces converge to yield but one reasonable course of action and those in which others (for example, health professionals) manipulate events (including withholding information) so that one has no choice. My dignity as a person is compromised in the latter case but not in the former, despite the fact that in both situations I may say that I have no choice. In the former case *I* still chose the one rational option. In the latter, I was a mere object acted upon.

Of course, there are times in some people's lives (e.g., periods of deep depression, drug-induced psychoses, or even moments of uncontrollable irrationality) when they lose the ability to make choices based on reasons. Tragically, some people have such severe mental impairment that they never achieve the capacity to work through and with a life-plan and thereby, to determine their own destiny. Young children have yet to develop these capacities. In all these cases, we would consider the person to be incompetent. Since competency is a necessary condition for applying the requirement of informed consent, it would not make sense to require it in these cases.

As was indicated before, the most frequent strategy for circumventing the requirement of informed consent is to claim that the client is not competent. To determine whether this is a legitimate move or is merely an evasive strategy, we must have a criterion or test for competency. From what we have said, the rough outline of such a test would be as follows: the person has the ability to work through and with a life-plan, i.e., has some sense of personal identity and some basic goals, aspirations, or values by which he or she chooses to live. The person has the ability to make choices on the basis of reasons and remains open to the claims of reason, so that upon hearing and considering additional reasons he or she could change his or her mind. Finally, the person is prepared to act on the basis of these choices and to take responsibility for them.

A word of caution is necessary in applying this criterion for competency. One must be able to put oneself in the other person's shoes, to think in terms of that person's values and general outlook on the world. For example, if a client believes in life after death and that accepting certain treatment (although medically beneficial) will jeopardize his chances for eternal bliss, it is quite reasonable for him to reject the treatment. A health professional may consider this worldview to be absurd and one she is not tempted to adopt. But that is irrelevant; the criterion must be applied relative to the client's life-plan and fundamental values. In the next section concerning paternalism we shall consider several such cases and argue that interference to prevent a client's choice in cases such as this is indefensible.

In many cases, by applying the competency test we will be able to determine either that a person is competent or is not. As with all such criteria, however, there will be borderline cases, such as the following case in which it is difficult to determine whether the person is competent (and, therefore, whether it is morally justifiable to go against her wishes and impose further treatment).

(F)

Mary Malone, a quarrelsome and despondent matron in her mid-fifties, was the chief clinical problem on the ward. She had admitted herself to the psychiatric ward of the private hospital in the depths of despair. Her husband had died four months earlier after a prolonged and agonizing series of operations for cancer. She had refused an invitation to live with her son, saying she believed that "my daughter-in-law doesn't want to have anything to do with me."

The diagnosis was acute, severe depression. Electroshock therapy was agreed upon by the two psychiatrists and the neurologist who examined her. She was given a careful explanation of the treatment and told that a series of shocks would be necessary. They would be very unpleasant, of which she was aware, but she agreed to the treatment. She said, "I really don't care what happens to me anymore." She readily signed the permission for the series.

On the morning of the first treatment she was given amobarital for sedation. At the instant of the shock she experienced a convulsion similar to a grand mal epileptic seizure. Two days later she was scheduled for a second treatment. That morning she was very anxious. She broke her fast, begging some food from another patient. The treatment had to be postponed until the next morning.

On that morning she made her stand. In a fit of anxious rage she screamed that she would have no further electroshock treatment. "That machine was torture," she yelled. "I won't let you touch me again." She leaped for the door, but it was locked. She turned to flee from the staff who had gathered around her. The psychiatrist tried to explain to her that the treatments would make her well again, and that even though they were unpleasant right now, they would be best for her in the long run. Every means of persuasion was used, but she was adamant.

In the staff meeting the arguments for continuing the therapy were heated: "Now that she has started the treatments, it would be a disaster to stop." "She really isn't enough in control of her faculties to refuse the treatment." "Certainly we cannot just release her." "I'm not giving her a choice at this point." "It is clear what is best for her even if she is too sick to understand." "We have a signed consent for the treatment." These arguments prevailed. Screaming and yelling, Mrs. Malone was dragged to the electroshock room by the nurses and attendants under the direction of the psychiatrist who was giving the treatment [Veatch, 1977, pp. 309–10].

Was Mary Malone competent when she signed herself into the hospital? Suppose that we determine that she was. Did she lose her ability to act with competence upon receiving the electroshock therapy and refusing further treatment? Clearly the question of competency is a complicated matter. In addition to relying on our own experience and understanding of people, we must rely on specialists, such as psychiatrists and psychiatric nurses, to determine whether the specific treatment (as seems likely) causes temporary loss of rationality, disorientation, and an increase in regressive behavior. If in fact this is the case, then the nurses in this case who restrained Ms. Malone and forced her to proceed with the treatment acted properly. Her incompetent state releases us from the requirement to obtain informed consent.

It is important to be clear about the fact that the question of a client's competency is not a moral issue. It is a factual matter best determined by people trained to recognize its presence or absence. Depending on what, in fact, is the case, we have certain moral duties toward the client or we do not. But deciding whether a client is competent is a prelude to making a moral judgment and not itself one.

Since the reason for insisting on informed consent before proceeding with any invasive treatment is the preservation and protection of individual self-determination, the exceptions to the rule are those cases in which self-determination is not possible—as in the above case in which (as we have assumed) the client is not competent.

We have seen that informed consent is a stringent requirement—one that, no matter how burdensome, must be satisfied in the treatment of all competent clients. We examined the elements of informed consent and considered the difficult issue of determining client competency. We warned against using the competency question as a way of circumventing the moral requirement of informed consent. On this issue, as with so many others, the nurse has a key role to play—one often complicated by the fact that not all members of the health team are working in concert.

When, If Ever, Is Coercion Permissible?

It is often alleged that *for the client's own good* decisions may be made that disregard or even oppose his or her own current inclinations or wishes. The doctrine that affirms that we are morally justified in acting against a person's freedom of choice in so doing to protect or advance that person's true or long-range interests is paternalism (acting as a parent toward another). In this section we shall examine when, if ever, paternalistic behavior is morally defensible. When, if ever, is a nurse or any other health professional morally justified in taking charge and disregarding a client's autonomy, setting aside the requirement of informed consent for reasons referring exclusively to the welfare, good, happiness, needs, interests, or values of the client who is being constrained?

For the sake of clarity, it is useful to distinguish between paternalistic grounds for constraint (the good of the person who is being constrained) and other grounds for constraint, (for example, self-defense or prevention of injury to another). Very different justifications are in order in the latter cases than in the former. We are likely to have far less difficulty defending our interference to stop one person from injuring another (including ourselves) than defending our interference to stop a person from injuring himself or herself. Our concern in this chapter is with defenses that can be given for paternalistic interference.

Anyone who wants to help another person in distress is likely to see the appeal of acting paternalistically. Health professionals in particular often feel that they have been thrust into the parent surrogate role, and to act paternalistically seems quite appropriate.

Consider, for example, the following case of a public health nurse:

(G)

In caring for an unwed mother and her child, the public health nurse was responsible for the health of the two clients. A social worker was assigned to work with the mother in relation to her provision for the child. If the unwed mother wished to give the child up and place it for adoption the law indicated she had a certain length of time in which to make her decision. After this length of time she must retain the care and legal responsibility for the child herself.

The public health nurse learned that the social worker had made an error in telling the young mother the length of time for a decision. The public health nurse felt it would be best for the mother to make her decision in the shorter length of time. She did not correct the information for the mother, because she thought that the mother could begin adjusting to her final decision more quickly with the earlier deadline [Tate, 1977, p. 37].

Here the public health nurse feels that the unwed mother is really better off if she is under an artifically shortened time constraint. Her long-range interests are better served by the imposition of a limitation on her current choices.

We can appreciate her desire to help and may be willing to concede that an earlier deadline would be beneficial to the client, yet the public health nurse's paternalistic behavior is not morally defensible. It presumes that the client is not able to make a rational decision, or at least is less able to do so than the nurse. But nothing in the account of the case establishes that. This seemingly admirable attitude fails to see that, for her own maturation and self-esteem, the client must not be prevented from taking full responsibility, must not be an object of benevolent manipulation. Had the nurse really respected the client's autonomy she would have informed her that she had more time to decide than the social worker erroneously indicated. In addition, she would have gone on to point out that there were good reasons for making the decision concerning adoption as early as possible.

Because we appreciate the nurse's genuine concern for the welfare of her client, we may be very reluctant to criticize her action. Yet if we consider this example as part of a much larger pattern of paternalistic practice—especially in the hospital setting—we can see the need to take a firm stand in protecting client autonomy. One of the greatest threats to a person who becomes a patient (here "patient" if more appropriate than "client") is that he or she will lose his or her autonomy.

The American Nurses' Association *Code of Ethics* has recognized the historical fact that patients occupy a dependent role with respect to health professionals and especially physicians. As we have seen, to express their concern that patients' not lose their autonomy and become passive objects of manipulation, they have used the term "client" rather than "patient" in their code. Of course, as everyone recognizes, the terminological change is not single-handedly going to counter-balance all the factors that contribute to client or patient dependence. Even with a terminological change, the client is sick, the health professional is well; the client is likely to lack knowledge, whereas the health professional has it; the client is a single individual, while the health professional is part of a vast institution and a network of other professionals.

Given the unequalness of the relationship and the client's strong need and desire for help, frequently he or she is quite ready to surrender some or even all of his or her autonomy, if that is what it takes to get relief. But autonomy is not something an adult happily or willingly gives up. The inequality of the relationship, as we saw in the previous section, puts the client who is trying to maintain as much autonomy as possible at a definite disadvantage relative to the health professional. This position of weakness gives the client no bargaining power.

Many who argue in favor of paternalism are not really concerned about a client's difficulties in preserving autonomy in the health care setting. They see the health professional's primary task as one of looking out for the best interests of the client, not as of protecting his or her autonomy. Once out of the hospital, they would argue, the client can again recover his or her autonomy. Dependency is seen as a price to be paid for good health care.

Nevertheless, not all who support some paternalistic actions need do so from a position of disregard for the fundamental value of maximal autonomy. We shall argue that there is room for a moderate position consistent with a deep concern for autonomy.

Let us look more closely at paternalism. It is a defense of dependency in a particular area of a person's life or at a particular time in his or her life. The health professional justifying his or her interventionist actions by appeal to the doctrine of paternalism is saying that it is permissible to take over the decision-making to disregard the person's autonomy in this area or at this particular time because to do so is in the client's best interest. Obviously, the viewpoint of this chapter is incompatible with the argument for paternalism, which claims that the duty to promote a client's best interests generally takes priority over the duty of noninterference and protecting another's autonomy. But it is a more complicated matter to determine whether any instances of paternalism may be compatible with the position of this chapter. Given the basic moral principles we have developed, as well as our discussion of the moral requirement of informed consent, our question must be: Would a health professional ever by justified in acting paternalistically?

If any cases can be justified, the most likely type of case would be one in which the client's decision will gravely, perhaps irreversibly, affect his or her own good. Examples include suicide, refusal of life-saving medical treatment, and choice of an unorthodox alternative treatment that clearly is not "medically indicated."

We shall examine two cases of refusal of life-saving medical treatment. They are written from the point of view of the involved nurse. The responses to the client's refusal of life-saving treatment are very different in the two cases.

(H)

Approximately 15 years ago, an elderly female patient, Ms. F., was admitted to the medical service of a hospital where I was employed. Among other problems, she was found to have a hemoglobin of 5 gms and, after further evaluation, the doctor ordered a type and crossmatch for five units of whole blood. Ordinarily, this should not have presented a problem, but in checking through her record, I discovered she was a Jehovah's Witness. When the doctor made his rounds later that day, I called his attention to Ms. F.'s religious preference. We discussed this at great length, noting that although she had many relatives, none of them had called her or written her, and no one had visited with her in 20 years. While the doctor and I were talking, he had written the order on her chart for her to have the first unit of blood. I told him I did not want to start the transfusion and he very emphatically stated that she was to have the blood and I was to start it. Ms. F. was not rational at this time and could not possibly object, but the doctor said to disguise the blood somehow in case she should become rational and put up a fuss. I asked him how you disguised blood, and he said that would be left up to me, just do it! I really had mixed emotions about transfusing this lady, but I had been thoroughly indoctrinated in the old school of nursing that the nurse was to be obedient and subservient to the doctor, so I started the unit of blood on the patient and hung a pillowcase over the top of the intravenous fluid stand to cover as much of the blood as possible. I did a lot of praying that none of her family would suddenly take an interest in her and visit during this time [Carroll and Humphrey, 1979, pp. 145–46].

(I)

A 39-year-old mother of a large number of children was admitted to the hospital with intense hemorrhaging. The family seemed very loving and caring for each other. But they were firm in their religious convictions which did not allow blood transfusions. After the doctor talked with her and her husband, he discontinued his order to give blood. He seemed so calm, but I was very upset about his decision. I felt he should have tried harder to get the family (all of whom were in on the decision, even the small children) to allow blood to be given. I let him know of my feelings and very calmly and patiently he sat down and told me that he did not have the right or authority to tamper with this family's religious convictions, and that he was not sure he could save her life with surgery and transfusions [Carroll and Humphrey, 1979, p. 155].

There can be no question that for anyone, especially someone trained as health professional, it would be very difficult to see someone die who could quite possibly be saved by a fairly routine medical procedure. For those who do not share the client's religious convictions, the resultant death would seem a waste. Yet if we respect the right of self-determination and give it the preeminence argued for in this essay, we must accept this outcome. We must agree that these clients have freely chosen to live their lives by the principles of the Jehovah's Witnesses. They have accepted as a fundamental doctrine the biblical injunction against eating blood, which they interpret as prohibiting blood transfusions. When a person truly adheres to religious values, these are the strongest and most central of his or her values. These provide the adherent with meaning and guidance for life. Decisions are made in conformity with the guidelines and priorities of the faith. A consequence of respect for client autonomy is that in cases such as these, in which there is no doubt that the client adheres to a religious view incompatible with the course of action medically indicated, one must refrain from imposing the medically indicated treatment on the client.

It may seem to follow from this conclusion that paternalistic intervention can never be morally justified. We must look carefully, however, and notice how these cases differ in a very significant way from other cases. In these cases the choice to forego treatment is consistent with the client's own basic values and commitments. We have difficulty with the choice, if we do, because we do not share the same values and commitments with the client. In other cases, such as the case of the woman refusing electroshock treatment after the procedure had been initiated (case F), we cannot be sure either that the decision is compatible with her basic values and commitments (although the initial decision to undergo treatment may have been) or that she is acting voluntarily at all. These differences, I shall argue, are crucial.

If we are going to defend paternalistic intervention in the Jehovah's Witness cases (cases H and I), we must argue that we are permitted to intervene to prevent another from doing an action *we* see as harmful to him, even when that person is acting of his or her own free will and is in full knowledge of the harm involved in his or her act. Such an argument fails to give the principle of autonomy its due. It allows a health professional to impose his or her values upon the client in situations in which the client's choice is unacceptable to the health professional (given the health professional's values). On the other hand, arguing that we may intervene and go against a person's current wishes in the following types of cases is defensible: (1) when it is clear that the person is not acting voluntarily (e.g., she is delirious, in shock, or under the influence of mind-altering medications or drugs); (2) when immediate action is necessary and the person is not adequately informed (e.g., does not know the adverse side-effects of the drug, or does not know that refusal of the treatment will result in a painful, prolonged death); and (3) when the person's choice is not compatible with his or her own best interests or fundamental values as he or she would define them, if thinking clearly.

Let us consider the reasons why paternalistic intervention is compatible with the position of this essay, and specifically the principle of autonomy in each of these types of cases.

1. We are not infringing upon one's autonomy if the person's actions are not voluntary. Only voluntary actions can be autonomous. Only preventing voluntary actions would interfere with another's self-determination. Hence, preventing another's nonvoluntary action for that person's own good is not incompatible with a strong affirmation of autonomy.

2. A person who is acting autonomously is acting rationally; that is, the person is open to reason and changing his or her mind if new conflicting evidence becomes available. If such a person, unbeknownst to him or her, is acting on clearly insufficient information and the *only* way to prevent adverse effects resulting from the action is to constrain that individual, this also would not be incompatible with the principle of autonomy. The person constrained would realize that the action he or she would have performed with misinformation or insufficient information would not have been an expression of self-determination. It would not have been the action that the actor or agent took it to be.

3. Great fear, depression, anger, a desire to get revenge, and so on, can lead us to act in ways that are not at all compatible with our own best interests and that are not really in accordance with our own actual preferences and desires. For example, imagine a young man jilted by his girlfriend, who feels that all is lost and attempts suicide by taking an overdose of sleeping pills. His various emotions, including depression and perhaps a desire to get revenge, we as observers may readily see, have clouded his vision. Although he cannot absorb it, we can see that all is not lost; there will be future joys; there will be other and perhaps

even better friendships. Were he able to see this unfortunate set-back in perspective, he could realize this as well; but for the moment he cannot. In cases such as this, interference and temporarily imposing our own will on another in no way violates the principle of self-determination. The *self* has not acted. Preventing the (in this case, irreversible) effects of the irrational action from overwhelming (here destroying) the individual, on the contrary, makes it possible for the self again to take stock and gain control of things.

We have argued that there are at least three types of situations in which paternalistic interference is justified, that is, is compatible with the position based on autonomy that has been developed in this essay. Given the compatibility of paternalistic intervention with the principle of autonomy, in these restricted situations, there are strong practical reasons to adopt a policy of paternalism as our way of responding to them. As Gerald Dworkin has argued:

Under certain conditions it is rational for an individual to agree that others should force him to act in ways in which, at the time of action, the individual may not see as desirable. If, for example, a man knows that he is subject to breaking his resolves when temptation is present, he may ask a friend to refuse to entertain his requests at some later stage [Dworkin, 1972, p. 76].

Paternalism, when it preserves or enables an individual to carry out his or her rational decisions and protects the person from irrational ones, not only is no threat to autonomy, it is a means of promoting it. It would seem reasonable then to adopt such a policy. As Dworkin says:

I suggest that since we are all aware of our irrational propensities, deficiences in cognitive and emotional capacities and avoidable and unavoidable ignorance it is rational and prudent for us to in effect take out "social insurance policies." We may argue for and against proposed paternalistic measures in terms of what fully rational individuals would accept as forms of protection [Dworkin, 1972, p. 77].

Dworkin continues:

Since we are all aware of the possibility of temporary states, such as great fear or depression, that are inimical to the making of well-informed and rational decisions, it would be prudent for all of us if there were some kind of institutional arrangement whereby we were restrained from making a decision which is (all too) irreversible [Dworkin, 1972, p. 81].

Dworkin is correct in arguing that it would be rational for us to adopt such a policy. Given that it is compatible with the ethical position we have developed and that it is a sensible view to hold, it offers us the best guidance for cases in which we must decide whether or not to engage in paternalistic action.

Our discussion has made clear what sort of cases do not allow paternalistic intervention (the Jehovah's Witness cases discussed) and the three general types of cases in which such intervention is permissible and perhaps required. But as we have seen with other guidelines and distinctions, there will always be borderline cases difficult to resolve. (Similarly, we may have a clear conception of the color red as well as of the color orange; we may be quite adept at distinguishing between them; but then we come across a color patch which we cannot be sure is red and orange. This does not mean that we have lost our ability to distinguish the colors or that there is no real distinction between them. It just means that we have come across a difficult borderline case.)

Let us look at one such case, a case of attempted suicide, and then compare it with a slightly different case.

(J)

During the many years that I have worked at this hospital, I have often been confronted with people who are depressed and have either attempted suicide or are verbally threatening to do so. During the first few years that I had to deal with these people, my opinion was that suicide was a sin and that a person should be prevented at all costs from inflicting this final act upon oneself. I have given drugs per doctor's order freely to such people and even physically restrained them. One incident that I shall never forget occurred some years ago. I was working on second shift by myself. I was responsible for 150 patients. Only another nurse in an adjoining building and a doctor on call and several attendants comprised the staff on duty. About 7:00 p.m. I was called to a ward which housed mostly middle-aged men who were more or less ready to be released from the hospital. When I arrived on the scene, the available attendants were surrounding a patient who was bleeding profusely from a wound in his lower right arm. He was swinging a chair at the attendants when they came close. Upon seeing me, he dropped the chair and began crying. The attendants pinned him to the floor and he began screaming, "Let me die." I immediately attempted to put direct pressure on his wound which was bleeding badly but he fought any attempt to stop the bleeding. After a struggle, I did manage to get the bleeding under control. The patient continued to cry and plead with me to let him die. We were surely a sight!—restraining a person on the floor with our white uniforms covered with blood. The patient had to be sedated before his wound could be sutured. Since then I have seen this man several times during the past four years. He has only been home several times during those years for short periods. He has rapidly deteriorated and now looks many years older than he is. He usually will speak and hold his arm up and announces in a loud voice, "She saved my life." There is no thanks in his voice, only the question "Why did you not let me die?" [Carroll and Humphrey, 1979, pp. 156-57].

At least in retrospect, the nurse feels that her action to save the client may have been wrong. But it is far from clear that intervention was not the morally right course. Consider the following case, in which it is clear that intervention is a violation of the client's autonomy. Comparing the two will help us to see which factors make the first case one that is difficult to decide.

(K)

A 60-year old man is brought to the emergency room. He is near death from an overdose of the pain-relieving drug Percodan. His private doctor is contacted and urges that everything be done to sustain life. Intensive resuscitation measures resulted in his life being saved. The man, who had been diagnosed two years prior as having bronchogenic carcinoma with multiple metastases to bone, suffered periodic seizures and required repeated aspiration and the instillation of nitrogen mustard. He had been taking Percodan daily for the relief of pain to little effect. Earlier that week he had spoken with the doctor and indicated that, having had two years to think about it, he just no longer had the will to live. He had discharged all his family responsibilities. The life that was left to him, as far as he was concerned, was no life at all. The doctor indicated that he could understand how difficult it must be but urged him to make the best of it.

In this case, the doctor's directive to use intensive measures to resuscitate the client is not justified. It is the doctor's inability to accept the client's conclusion rather than the client's irrationality or lack of information or inability to act freely that is the determining factor in this decision. Nor, in this case, can there be much reason to think that the suicide attempt is a cry for help rather than an action intended by the client to provide a release from life.

None of these things are certain one way or the other in the first case. Some aspects of the case point one way, and others point the other. These ambiguous situations, unfortunately, tend to be more prevalent than the clear-cut ones. A health professional does not have the luxury of standing around debating the pros and cons. Action is required. A policy for ambiguous cases is needed. From all we have said, it would seem that the best action-guide would be one of intervention in such cases: the action is irreversible, it may be a cry for help, it may be an irrational act. The danger, of course, is that the policy will be misused as a rationalization for intervention in clear cases, such as case K. Honesty in applying the principle is essential.

We conclude this section on paternalism with another troubling thought: sometimes being a client advocate and respecting a person's right to self-determinism as well as acting on the general prohibition against paternalism, which we have defended, may require a nurse to counteract the paternalistic practices of others on the health care team. Following is such a case:

(L)

I had worked for several nights in an Intensive Care Unit with a woman who had metastatic cancer. At some point during her illness she refused further chemotherapy and told her family she wanted to stay at home without further treatment until the end came. However, it became increasingly difficult for her to breathe and one evening a family member took her to the emergency room. She was placed on a respirator without the doctor knowing the basis of the problem. With proper oxygenation, her brain functioned well and she was furious with everyone. Her arms were restrained and of course she couldn't talk, but still she begged with her eyes and hands. I had read her chart, talked with her family, knew the doctor regretted putting her on the respirator but wouldn't take her off. I tried to reason with her and explained her lungs wouldn't function sufficiently without the machine. She understood this but had reached that point when life was unbearable. So, one night when I finished cleaning her, I didn't secure her arm restraints well. She extubated herself and died that night [unpublished case from Pecorino].

Must the Nurse Always Tell the Truth?

From personal experience I would say that the patients who aren't told about their terminal illness have so many verbal and mental questions unanswered that many will begin to realize that their illness is more serious than they're being told. . . . Nurses care for these patients twenty-four hours a day compared to a doctor's daily brief visit, and it is the nurse many times that the patient will relate to, once his underlying fears become overwhelming. . . . This is difficult for us nurses because being in constant contact with patients we can see the events leading up to this. The patient continually asks you, "Why isn't my pain decreasing?" or "Why isn't the radiation treatment easing the pain?" [letter from Mary Barrett, *Boston Globe*, 16 Nov. 1976].

The nurse is caught in the middle on the issue of truth-telling. Sometimes telling the truth may seem to the nurse to be the only moral course of action, yet the physician may not want the truth told. Other times the nurse, while wanting to be forthright, may not be certain how much the doctor has told the client and feel that she or he should not go beyond the doctor's explanation. Or it may be the case that both doctor and nurse agree that telling the truth would cause an already sick client avoidable anguish. Yet as client advocates, they may feel they owe the client candor. Some nurses may find it distressing to be candid with clients with poor prognoses but question the morality of not telling the truth in order to avoid unpleasantness. In still other cases (for example, treatment using placebos) deception may be an element of the treatment plan. To say, "Here's a placebo (a sugar pill); take two every four hours and you'll feel better," obviously would not do. In yet other cases, the health team simply may not know what is wrong with a client or what course of treatment to follow. Since sharing these facts with the client may be thought to undermine his or her confidence in the health team, which in turn may negatively affect his or her chances of recovery, withholding the information or even lying to the client may appear to be the morally proper course.

We can all agree that, generally speaking, one ought to tell the truth. It is easy to agree to such universal and vague propositions. Yet pointing to such agreement is not an empty exercise. It commits us to more than we may first think. Being willing to make a presumption in favor of truth-telling, it follows that the burden of justification is on the person who engages in deception. Anyone engaging in deception must be able to offer a defense.

As the issue of truth-telling is confronted by the nurse, the dangers of not telling the truth are clearly evident. But just as clear is the fact that, in certain situations, the freedom to withhold information and to deceive clients seems necessary in order to do what one must as a good nurse. In some situations, telling the truth appears to be inflicting avoidable anguish, dashing another's hopes, shortening another's life, or radically limiting the treatment options.

In this chapter we shall discuss the issue of truth-telling and see if we can provide clarification and some guiding principles. After briefly examining current practice regarding truth-telling among health professionals, we shall see what principles can be derived from the basic position that has been developed in this work. Using these principles, we shall consider several cases.

At least until recently the most common answer to the question, "When, if ever, may a health professional deceive his or her client?" has been the paternalistic one. That is, deception, even lying, has been thought to be justified when (in the judgment of the health professional) it is in the best interests of the client. On this view, the guiding principle for deciding whether to tell the truth is "Do no harm." If truth-telling is considered by the physician to be harmful to the client, it should be avoided. If lying is seen by the physician as harmful, he or she should not lie. The prevalence of this paternalistic view is probably the reason most professional codes—beginning with the Hippocratic Oath—omit mention of any duty to tell the truth or to be honest with one's clients. In recent years, however, partly because of the strength of the consumer movement in health care and the popularity of such documents as the Patient's Bill of Rights, professional groups, including the American Medical Association, have begun to rethink their stance on this issue (see Veatch, 1980, p. 17).

The change of position in recent years on the part of physicians is evidenced in two studies—in 1961 and in 1977—concerning what to tell cancer patients. The 1961 study reported that 90 percent of the responding physicians had a preference for not telling cancer patients the diagnoses. The 1977 study of physicians had 97 percent of those responding indicating a preference for telling the diagnosis to a cancer patient (*New York Times*, 26 February 1979).

Some have speculated that the major reason for the change is the threat of malpractice suits. The argument is that physicians recognize that they can minimize their liability when they transmit information to the client. It puts the client in a position of responsibility. A less-cynical explanation (the one I favor) is the increasing awareness among physicians of the desirability of client autonomy and of the requirements for maintaining client autonomy. Surely, physicians can recognize that the arguments leading to the conclusion that informed consent is required (as we discussed above) also lead to the conclusion that we must make a strong presumption in favor of telling the truth.

Let us see what position on truth-telling is most consistent with the position we have developed in this book. We have argued that our most basic duty is that of respecting other persons (as well as ourselves) as persons. The duty of truth-telling is part of the respect we owe to persons. For instance, I fail to show you the respect you are due if, because I feel it would be a mistake for you to buy it, I tell you that an item in the store which you want is priced at $75 when I know it is priced at $45. I am treating you as an object to be manipulated, because I do not see you as someone whose desires, ends, hopes, and aspirations must be honored. Were you later to discover that I deceived you in this way, you would have grounds for complaint, even if you then agreed that you were better off without the item. Had I, on the other hand, informed you of my belief that purchasing the item would be a mistake and then given you the reasons for my belief, I would have been respecting your autonomy and treating you as a rational person. In this case, another acceptable alternative would have been to say nothing at all. But if I choose to speak, the respect I owe to you requires that I communicate what I believe to be the case. (The alternative of saying nothing is not always an acceptable one. As we shall see, one's role or relationship to the other person may actually make to say nothing a deceptive communication, or the situation may not allow one to remain silent.)

The close relationship between the requirements of truth-telling and informed consent is evident. Both are based on the principle of autonomy. Consent cannot express autonomy, as we saw in the first section of this chapter, unless it is informed. Truthfulness is the clearest means to being informed. We have established that health professionals have a duty to protect their clients' autonomy and to inform them of their diagnoses, prognoses, and so on. The duty of veracity (telling the truth) then arises from the same source: the principle of autonomy or respect for persons.

We saw in our discussions of informed consent and paternalism that each of these duties is stringent; yet there are situations in which the respect for persons upon which they are based can be better served by violating the duties. Similarly here, the duty of veracity is a stringent one based on the fundamental principle of autonomy. If we find that there are cases in which it is morally permissible or even morally obligatory to set the duty aside, they will be cases in which lack of candor, deception, or perhaps even lying promote clients' autonomy better than telling the truth. Deception that does not promote client autonomy is morally unacceptable.

The cases that follow demonstrate the unacceptability of deception that does not promote autonomy. The first is a sad case describing the sense of being wronged felt by a client when she or he has been deceived—even when the motives for the deception are honorable.

Cheryl was a student nurse who entered the General Programme in 1972. Some months after she entered the programme and several attacks of tonsillitis, Cheryl was diagnosed as having acute lymphatic leukaemia. Her parents were told of the situation and were specifically requested by the consultant, as was the entire nursing staff, not to divulge the diagnosis to Cheryl.

Owing to her illness Cheryl quickly dropped behind in her class. Recognizing that the hospital environment was not in the best interest of her precarious health, employment outside the hospital was suggested. After she entered her first remission, she found a position she liked as a secretary in a commercial enterprise.

Cheryl maintained reasonable health under a specific anti-mitotic regime. At approximately five- to six-month intervals, she required one or two days of hospitalization to have the blood content and volume restored to normal limits. On each occasion for the first two years, she greeted the staff warmly and seemed to enjoy the break in her usual routine of living that hospital treatment required.

During the third year of her illness Cheryl's attitude to the staff altered considerably and the staff found it increasingly uncomfortable to be in her presence. She rarely asked questions and withdrew from any social interaction. The periods of hospitalization altered gradually so that, three years after the diagnosis was established, Cheryl was admitted with a large necrosing area extending from the perineum into the buttock and enlarging rapidly.

The consultant caring for Cheryl maintained a rigorous system for infection control of his hospitalized leukaemic patients. They were segregated in single rooms and neither staff nor visitors were allowed into the rooms without paper caps, gowns, masks and overshoes.

As Cheryl passed into the terminal phase of her illness, the nursing staff asked repeatedly for the medical staff to discuss with her her ultimate prognosis. Had this been done, it was believed that the charade of possible recovery would have been dropped between Cheryl and her family allowing them at least the possibility of open expression [Tate, 1977, pp. 29-30].

In situations such as this one, deception proves to be ineffectual. But even if it were effectual, the arrogant (even if well-meaning) manipulation of the client is a direct affront to self-determination. This case is similar to so many in which evasive techniques are practiced. We really have no good reason to think that the client is unable to exercise control over his or her own life, and we project our own difficulties of facing the tragedy upon the victim.

In the following case there is more substantial ground for questioning whether the client can (at the moment) respond rationally to the truth. If it is evident that the client cannot, the major objection to deception, namely, its undermining of autonomy, is not applicable. (If the client cannot act autonomously—that is, does not have autonomy—it is not possible to take it away from him or her.) The crucial question is: Is the client capable of autonomous action? Answering this question is difficult and frequently may require assistance from experts (e.g., psychiatrists). All too often, it is a judgment we are eager to make in order to minimize our own discomfort and uneasiness. If we too hastily determine that a client is incapable of autonomous action and base our intervention upon it, as in the case below, the client will sense that he or she has been wronged.

Recently, whilst [I was] working on evening duty in a small country hospital as Sister-in-charge, the victims of a road accident were admitted to my ward. The driver of the vehicle, which had left the road and overturned spilling the children out, was the children's mother. She and her four children had all been personally known to me for some time.

The two middle children, both boys, were nearly scalped, but had their flaps sutured in place and made uneventful recoveries. The smallest daughter eventually completely lost the use of one arm. The eldest child, a girl of thirteen, suffered severe head injuries and died shortly after admission. The mother suffered contusions and abrasions, however, the greatest area of concern was her hysterical mental state in regard to the injuries to her children when she was driving the car.

Despite tranquilizers, this mental condition did not improve until she was heavily sedated later in the night. Throughout the evening her greatest concern was for her eldest daughter who had apparently been the quietest at the scene of the accident and whom she instinctively felt was in the most danger.

Because of my position on the ward and the fact that I was personally known to her, she constantly entreated me to inform her of the children's condition. When it became obvious that the daughter was about to die, I asked the doctor what I should tell the mother as he was busy in the operating theatre and could not speak to her himself.

The woman's husband lived some distance away and could not be contacted for several hours, and I was instructed that, because of her distress, the doctor would prefer to inform her in the company of her husband, and until that time I was to re-assure her at all costs.

Over the next few hours, during my ministrations to her, she repeatedly queried me about the children and particularly the eldest daughter. It went strongly against my conscience to have to look her in the eye and repeat a lie of such magnitude.

She was finally sedated and early next morning when her husband and doctor told her the real news her distress was heralded with the cry "Why did she lie to me?"

Through various circumstances, I have not seen her since but her husband has told me that, although she understood my instructions had come from her doctor, she felt my behavior and his had amounted to unethical interference. She no longer considers me a friend. Try as I will, I cannot believe that my action in this case was ethical [Tate, 1977, pp. 31-33].

The principles advanced in this essay support the nurse in her judgment that the deception is morally indefensible. Since the burden of proof is on the individual who chooses not to tell the truth, we need a much stronger defense of the evasive and deceptive behavior than a vague reference to her "hysterical mental state." (Who wouldn't be "hysterical" at a time like this? Wouldn't we really have our doubts about someone who took it all in stride?) Intuitively, these are the kinds of cases in which deception, including lying, seems defensible. But such a defense has not been presented in this particular case.

Several distinctions must be made, however, to make it clear why the action taken in this case is wrong, while rather similar action in seemingly similar (although actually different) circumstances may be judged morally defensible. Using these distinctions, we shall compare this case with several variations on it.

Being reserved or "close-mouthed" or withholding information must be distinguished from being deceptive. We may feel that we would be wronging another person by deceiving him or her but (quite correctly) feel no obligation to apprise him or her of a situation or of certain facts or of our beliefs. Suppose, for example, in contrast to the actual case, that the client does not ask about the condition of her eldest daughter. Or suppose that she does ask but you ignore the question and she does not ask it again. In these cases, you are not deceiving her. You simply are not volunteering any information. You are being reserved. Such behavior can be distinguished from deceiving a client: for example, acting as if everything is fine to provide a basis for a false conclusion about the situation, or telling her that you do not know how the daughter is (when you do know), or saying that she is out of danger.

Whether the distinction between withholding information and being deceptive is one that makes a *moral* difference depends on the expectations of the parties in the relationship. For example, suppose that the client reasonably expects that he will be apprised of any untoward findings from a battery of tests he has undergone. The health professionals decide (for the client's own good) not to inform him about the findings and his bad prognosis. Since the implicit premise of the relationship is that no news is good news, withholding the information is morally equivalent to telling a lie. Whether we withhold the information or give him false information we are misleading him; in so doing, we are restricting his autonomy. In contrast, when there is no expectation that information will be volunteered, withholding it does not constitute an infringement upon another's autonomy. In such cases, the distinction between withholding information and being deceptive is one that makes a moral difference. Given the current strong emphasis on informed consent and full disclosure, the health care contexts in which there is no expectation that information will be volunteered continue to diminish.

We must also make distinctions concerning ways of being deceptive. Intuitively, we feel that being evasive is often more easily defended than is lying. Generally speaking, lying to clients—telling them what one believes to be false in order to deceive them—deprives them of the chance to make genuine decisions about their lives. Unless one can clearly demonstrate that the client is unable to act rationally (e.g., is incompetent) or that for some other reason the lie in question does not deprive the individual of the chance to make an autonomous choice, the lie is morally indefensible. One cannot as categorically condemn evasiveness (with the intent to deceive), however. In being evasive one may be intentionally deceiving another, but one is acting with a certain amount of restraint in that one is not lying. From one's actions or statements one expects that the person who is the target of the deception will draw a false conclusion. Yet that false conclusion is not itself stated. It is up to the person deceived to draw that conclusion. Hence, the person being deceived is not merely a recipient of false information (which it is reasonable to presume is true), as is often the case with lying, but is, on the contrary, at least to a certain extent an active participant in the deception. He or she need not draw the conclusion that goes beyond the statement made (Ellin, 1981, p. 4). Being deceptive through evasion is not as forceful an attack on autonomy as is being deceptive through lying. The restraint of evasive deception is at least a concession to the importance of autonomy, whereas the willingness to lie reveals complete disregard for the rationality and autonomy of the other.

Using the distinctions we have just made, we have a range of strategies open to us, from candor (full disclosure), to withholding relevant information, to deception through evasion, to deception through lying. As we move across the continuum from candor to lying we increase the effectiveness of the means for hiding the truth, but we also increase the impediments to autonomous rational choice. The image of a window is useful here. Candor can be compared to a clear glass that allows the full light of day to pass through. As we move along the continuum and begin withholding information, we are darkening the glass. We are adding impediments to the passing of light. Lying is a fully darkened glass that allows no light to pass through. In this analogy, light is information. In being evasive and especially in lying, we intervene and alter the information reaching the client (either by withholding some part of it or by distorting it).

Suppose that we modify the case of the accident victim so that, if relayed, the information about her daughter's well-being would cause her to lose her small bit of rational control. Here we have a paradigm case for withholding the truth and even for using deception if necessary. But granted the assumption that this or any other client is unable to deal with the truth and that thus it ought not to be disclosed to him or her, we should move no further along the continuum from candor to lying than is necessary. We should take as few liberties as possible. For example, if being evasive can prevent the truth from being known when it should not be known, lying cannot be justified. Only when the less-extreme strategies fail would lying be defensible. Just as paternalism can sometimes be justified because it is the best means for preserving autonomy, so too can deception. But paternalism and deception are strategies of last resort. One must consider all other less-extreme alternatives and, where possible, adopt them even if they sometimes require more time, energy, or ingenuity. A health professional using the extreme measures must be prepared to demonstrate that less-drastic means were inadequate.

If we adopt the principle of minimum movement along the continuum from candor to lying, we are likely to conclude that in the health care arena we have had a tendency to condone deception, including lying, far too readily. Without a clear understanding of the various steps along the continuum and without an unambiguous demand that a justification be provided for each step, deceptive practices have become commonplace and are frequently engaged in simply as a matter of course. The distinctions and principles presented should help us to avoid these pitfalls.

Not only is the tendency to engage in deceptive practices morally unacceptable, it is also ill advised. The lack of candor and, especially, deception undermine relationships of trust—relationships that are necessary for fruitful interaction and cooperation. If the traditional confidence and trust found in the health professional–client relationship is undermined, one of the primary sources of healing and comfort will be lost.

Some writers have claimed that the history of medicine can best be characterized as the history of the placebo effect: the well-documented psychological phenomenon that even seriously ill clients' conditions improve through the attention, medication (even if only a sugar pill), or treatment (whatever it be) given by health professionals *in whom the client trusts* (see Evans, 1974). We know today that many of the potions and pills prescribed in the past did not have the pharmacologic effects they were thought to have, yet frequently they provided relief. The one constant that seems to have led to the relief these clients experienced is trust. Today, even with more effective treatments, trust remains a commodity of great value—one we must not squander.

The placebo effect—operative in relationships of trust—provides the basis for the effectiveness of placebos (defined in Stedman's Medical Dictionary as "an indifferent substance, in the form of a medicine, given for the suggestive effect"). The use of placebos adds a further dimension to the issues of candor and deception. As mentioned above, one cannot effectively administer placebos by telling the client, "Here are some placebos or sugar pills. Take these every four hours." The placebo effect (i.e., their effectiveness) would be lost. This points out the paradox of placebo therapy: it works only if it is administered in a context of trust. Yet, with the exception of carefully worked out situations, administration of placebos requires objectionable deception. If the person in whom I trust is willing to deceive me, is my trust misplaced? For trust to be properly placed shouldn't the person be trustworthy, not deceitful? Trust and deceit are an unstable mixture.

Despite the clear dangers to the relationship of trust and the moral problems entailed by the use of placebos, their successful use in the therapeutic context (not to mention their use in experimentation, which raises a different set of issues) provides the health professional with many reasons to want to use placebos. Placebos have been effective on clients suffering from conditions that include postoperative pain, angina pectoris, and the common cold. For the client who demands unneeded medication, a placebo can be very effective without risking the possible negative side-effects of medication that contains active ingredients. A placebo can be used effectively when physicians are uncertain about the diagnosis and are running additional tests but want to offer something to the client in the meantime.

We must ask, however, whether these benefits are sufficient to risk the loss of trust that may result from placebo use. George Heidrich, writing in a recent issue of *RN*, thinks they are not. "The placebo response is based on the patient's trust of the caregivers and it is very dangerous to do anything that may destroy that trust. The temporary relief a patient may get from a placebo is not worth the loss of faith he'll experience if he finds out you've fooled him" (Heidrich, 1980, p. 37). The placebo is a dangerous weapon. What is gained by using it can easily be lost. Use of placebos must not only meet the objection that it is deceptive but also that the inherent risks are worth taking.

The best way of meeting these objections would be to devise ways of minimizing the elements of deception and risk. That is, we must find ways to administer placebos which do not involve morally objectionable deception and the risk of a loss of trust. This may not always be possible. Nevertheless, frequently some ingenuity will reveal ways to do it. An example follows:

Suppose a postmenopausal woman came to me determined to get estrogen for her hot flashes, vasomotor symptoms, and mood changes. I could explain that I'm worried about the possible cancer-causing role of estrogen; and that while the drug may work well for the hot flashes and vasomotor symptoms, it hasn't been shown to do much for mood. Then I'd tell her that the mind is a powerful thing and we may be able to fool it into relieving her symptoms. "I'll give you estrogen for four weeks and a placebo for four weeks—you won't know which is which—and we'll see if we can relieve the symptoms with the least possible risk" [Sandroff, 1980].

The strategy devised here provides the key to the moral use of the placebo in therapeutic contexts. The client's rationality and autonomy are not ignored. The client agrees to remain ignorant about certain aspects of the treatment plan. With this prior agreement, the health professional runs no risk of a loss of confidence due to the lack of disclosure of the precise use of the placebo.

If clients are informed that the human being is a very complex organism and that we understand little about how the mind influences the body, pain sensation, healing processes, and so on, and (substitute here whatever explanatory theory you accept) that administering placebos may be a way of stimulating the nervous system to release endorphins (body-produced painkillers) and other helpful chemicals, clients can give prior agreement to the use of placebos along with other medication. In this way the deception necessary for effective administration of placebos does not violate the respect due to the person. His or her autonomy and rationality have been given proper regard. In those cases in which the person truly is unable to act autonomously and rationally, of course consultation and client participation will not be possible. But in these cases, since their lack of autonomy makes it impossible to remove it (through deception or any other means), the usual moral constraints concerning truth-telling do not apply. One must act on behalf of the client and decide for him or her with the hope that eventually rationality will be restored.

When, If Ever, May Confidentiality Be Breached?

Whereas professional codes of ethics have tended to have a minimal interest in truth-telling, they have strongly emphasized the importance of the confidentiality of the health professional–client relationship. Beginning with the ancient Hippocratic Oath and extending to present-day professional codes, the duty to maintain confidences entrusted to one in the course of medical attendance has been affirmed. The World Medical Association International Code, for example, is unyielding on this demand, claiming that the physician owes his or her client "absolute secrecy on all information which has been confided to him." Most other codes allow for exceptions in special situations, such as when the law of the state in which one is practicing requires revealing the information, or when divulging the information is necessary in order to protect the welfare of the individual or of others (the community).

Two kinds of legal protection of the principle of health professional–client confidentiality have been adopted by many states: (a) positive protection—legal sanctions that can be applied against health professionals who reveal confidential information acquired in the course of treatment—and (b) negative protection—statutes that exempt health professionals from the obligation to testify in court concerning what has been learned in the client–health professional relationship. (These statutes establish that communications between health professionals and clients are "privileged communications.")

Since health professionals in their codes of ethics have almost unanimously expressed their support for the confidentiality principle and since the people through their legislators have supported legal enforcement of it, no defense of the principle may seem necessary. Yet there are many times when a health professional may question the validity of the principle. In practice many situations arise in which it is difficult to maintain confidentiality, and one may feel that it ought to be breached. Thus, it is important to determine why we should have a rule concerning confidentiality, exactly what must be kept confidential, whether there are exceptions to the rule, how far the circle of confidentiality extends (e.g., if it includes all other health professionals and the patient's family), and whether the principle takes priority over other duties (such as the duty to tell the truth or the duty to prevent harm). These are the issues we shall examine in this section.

There are at least three interrelated reasons for maintaining a strong principle of confidentiality: (1) The respect owed to the client requires that the health professional preserve confidences. (2) If prospective clients did not have the assurance of confidentiality, they might not be willing to seek help for many of their problems. (3) There is an implied promise of confidentiality inherent in the health professional–client relationship. We shall examine each of these reasons, beginning with the second.

Many people would think twice about going for treatment and might even prefer to suffer than to risk having certain embarrassing or intimate personal facts become public knowledge. Reticence on the part of clients when questions are asked in the course of diagnoses and treatment would undoubtedly make these processes more difficult and interfere with their effectiveness. I suspect that from the beginning this practical consideration has played a large role in convincing health professionals of the need for a confidentiality principle. This also helps explain the prominence of the principle in the codes. It was important to let the public know that the professional groups were strongly committed to confidentiality.

Once the confidentiality constraint is in place (i.e., is established as a practice), maintaining it becomes a moral issue, namely, that of keeping agreements. If a professional group and the professionals in it have publicly stated that they will maintain confidentiality, this is the premise upon which their clients seek their services. Failure to keep confidences then is to renege on a commitment made.

Both of these considerations support adherence to the constraint of confidentiality. From the perspective of this essay, however, the crucial support for the principle is the first reason, namely, the fact that respect for persons as persons requires protecting the clients' privacy, which in turn entails preserving confidentiality.

The principle of the confidentiality of the health professional–client relationship is based on the right of privacy, which, as we shall see, is entailed by the principle of autonomy. Privacy is an element of autonomy. As Professor Richard Wasserstrom has stated:

> What it is to be a person carries with it . . . the idea of the existence of a core of thoughts and feelings that are the person's alone. If anyone else could know all that I am thinking or perceive all that I am feeling except in the form I choose to filter and reveal what I am and how I see myself—if anyone could, so to speak, be aware of all this at will I might cease to have as complete a sense of myself as a distinct and separate person as I have now. A significant, if not fundamental, part of what it is to be an individual person is to be an entity that

is capable of being exclusively aware of its own thoughts and feelings [Wasserstrom, 1976, p. 113].

It is useful to focus on the need for privacy both to shed greater light on the principle of autonomy itself and to clarify the moral source of the confidentiality principle. Wasserstrom asks us to imagine a setting in which virtually everything one does is recorded and known to others. It would be difficult for individuals who are the objects of such scrutiny to retain a sense of self, a sense of individuality and autonomy. It would also be difficult for those doing the monitoring to continue to retain a sense of the subjects as persons rather than objects.

Certain units (e.g., the intensive care unit) in the hospital are very much the settings Wasserstrom asks us to imagine. We can see how quickly the hospital setting can undermine the moral standing of both client and professional.

Patients, and especially patients in hospitals, are observed, monitored, checked and the information obtained thereby routinely and regularly recorded in accordance with notions of institutional regularity, thoroughness and convenience. . . . [I]t will . . . be difficult for a patient to preserve his or her sense of autonomy and individuality. In this environment it will be easy for those of the institution who are not patients to see themselves as different in important respects from the patients. They are not continually under scrutiny; the patients as objects are [Wasserstrom, 1976, p. 114].

The moral concern for privacy requires constant vigilance against unnecessary monitoring, examining, and questioning of clients. Although they are for the client's welfare, we have seen how they can undermine his or her most fundamental welfare, namely, his or her standing as a person.

Concern to honor the confidentiality of the client usefully focuses on divulging to others the information obtained in the course of treatment. Yet this concern is only the second half of the problem. The first half is obtaining more information from the client than is required. Especially when close monitoring is essential, it must be done with the utmost regard for preserving as much of the respect for persons as possible. Health professionals must be aware that uncritically using ever more-sophisticated diagnostic and monitoring equipment is a serious threat to the dignity of both client and health professional. As we take advantage of the new technology, we must not lose sight of the pitfalls.

Now let us turn to the issue of divulging confidential information. The reason we must make a strong presumption against the health professional doing so is derived from the right to privacy just discussed. In a classic essay on the right to privacy, Samuel Warren and

Louis Brandeis wrote in 1890 that the common law secured "to each individual the right of determining, ordinarily, to what extent his thoughts, sentiments, and emotions shall be communicated to others" (Walters, 1974, p. 171). Common law grants people this right because it is essential to maintaining the respect for autonomy upon which common law is based. The right to privacy places the power of disclosure in the hands of the individual. If the individual wishes to disclose any information concerning his or her health or attitudes or actions, that is his or her prerogative. If he or she authorizes disclosure of information, then doing so is not a breach of confidence. But disclosure without such authorization is *prima facie* wrong (i.e., in need of justification to demonstrate that keeping the confidence violates some other, more-stringent duty).

Contemporary defenders of the right to privacy frequently appeal to a model of the person as a complex entity with different needs for privacy, depending upon the area of one's life and one's relationship to those with whom the information may be shared.

In the center is the "core self," which shelters the individual's "ultimate secrets"—"those hopes, fears, and prayers that are beyond sharing with anyone unless the individual comes under such stress that he must pour out these ultimate secrets to secure emotional release." . . . [T]he next largest circle contains intimate secrets which can be shared with close relatives or confessors of various kinds. Successively larger circles are open to intimate friends, casual acquaintances, and finally to all observers [Walters, 1974, p. 171].

When clients subject themselves to medical treatment or place themselves under the care of a health professional, they share detailed information that may include innermost secrets of the heart. Out of necessity the health professional is admitted into the inner circle—a circle into which close friends of the client may have been denied admission. Clearly this makes the client vulnerable.

To see how wrong it would be freely to share this information with anyone else, consider a familiar character from life and fiction, the drunken husband who talks freely about his wife's secret fears, foibles, and fantasies. Because of the love and trust she has given to him, she is vulnerable and at his mercy. He, in his drunken disregard for her privacy, is treating her merely as an object. Whether he intends it or not, he is disregarding her dignity as a person and is exhibiting a profound moral deficiency. Although the context and motives for divulging confidential information are very different for health professionals than for our reprobate husband, the presumption of preserving confidences hold equally for all.

With the principle of confidentiality we again have a situation comparable to that with the other principles examined in this chapter (such as truth-telling and the prohibition against paternalism). We must make a strong presumption in favor of maintaining confidentiality, and only very strong reasons will be sufficient to outweigh its demands. The types of reasons that are sufficiently weighty are the conflicting requirements of other duties. In the course of everyday practice the nurse faces many such conflicts, a few samples of which we shall examine below.

Consider the following three types of situations in which, we shall argue, conflicting obligations provide sufficient ground to justify setting aside the confidentiality principle.

1. Generally speaking, confidentiality may be breached when maintaining a confidence is incompatible with maintaining the client's own true autonomy. (The discussion here ties in closely with the earlier discussion of paternalism.) Examples would be cases of clients in temporary fits of depression or anger, threatening to kill themselves, or to do some irrational act that will almost certainly destroy their prospects for full, autonomous lives. An illustration is a client who is being treated for a back injury. Although the prognosis is good, the treatment plan requires time and strenuous physical therapy. The client is in considerable pain. The ordeal causes him to become depressed and to lose patience with further treatment. During a conversation with the nurse, he states that he has decided upon suicide, the only solution he can see to his problem. As soon as he voices his plan, he asks the nurse to remain silent about his intentions. Being convinced that the only way she can be sure of preventing the suicide is to alert the next shift of nurses as well as the client's physician, she breaches the confidence. (This example is a modification of a case we discussed earlier.) She feels that her course of action is justified because maintaining the confidence is not the best way of protecting the client's real autonomy. Paternalistically she feels (quite correctly) that concern for the client's autonomy is best served by breaking this confidence.

The following is another example of a nurse being convinced that other duties to the client supersede her duty to maintain a confidence.

A young unmarried woman was admitted to the hospital with excessive uterine bleeding, which she explained was connected with her monthly period. She stated that this had occurred several times over the course of the past year and was of great concern to her.

A student nurse, of the approximate age of the patient, was caring for her the day after admission. The patient told the student that she was certain she was pregnant and had taken some medications which she had been told would bring about an abortion. She did not want anyone, even the doctor, to know about this. She asked the student nurse not to tell anyone, particularly the doctor.

The student nurse knew she should not reveal information given by the patient in confidence. However, she felt the proper treatment for the patient could not be carried out unless the doctor knew all the related facts on the patient's history. The student told the entire story to the doctor. The doctor then proceeded to talk with the patient phrasing his questions in such a way that the patient eventually told the doctor the same information herself. The doctor was then able to prescribe the appropriate treatment and still not reveal the breach of confidence [Tate, 1977, p. 21].

In both of these cases the duty to protect the client's autonomy leads the nurse to set aside the otherwise binding duty of confidentiality. These cases do not demonstrate that the duty to keep confidences is not generally binding, but they quite clearly show that it is a duty that can be superseded. The reason for this is the same as with the other duties we have discussed in this chapter: it is a *derived* duty (arising from the basic duty of respect for persons).

These cases raise the issue of the scope of confidentiality. In the cases cited, the client expected the circle of confidentiality to be drawn around the nurse herself. In many other contexts the circle will be wider to include, for example, all health professionals involved with the case. It is not always evident who the participants consider to be in the circle of confidentiality. This is a crucial issue. If we are not clear about it, we do not know whether we are faced with the question of violating a confidence. If the person with whom I want to share this information is in the circle, my telling her will not be a breach of confidentiality. Not being clear about the scope of confidentiality can also provide one with an easy excuse when a confidence has unjustifiably been broken. I will say, "I didn't know I was not supposed to tell *him*."

The scope of confidentiality depends in part upon conventions that have arisen and related expectations. In the cases under consideration (as also is frequently the case), it is explicitly stated. When the question of the scope is unclear, efforts must be made to clarify it. Whether family members should be considered within the circle of confidentiality is a problem frequently faced by nurses. Clearly, this varies in accordance with the closeness of the family and the type of confidential information. When possible the client is the one who should make the determination. The nurse as client advocate should facilitate that choice.

2. Generally speaking, confidentiality may be breached when maintaining a confidence is incompatible with the rights of an innocent third party. The classic example is the "battered child." Suppose a physician or nurse discovers evidence of abuse in the course of treating

an injured child. Generally speaking, as we have seen, what is learned in the course of treatment is to remain confidential, yet that comes into conflict with duties we have toward the vulnerable child. To assure that in practice the duties toward the victim be given greater weight, most states in the United States require health professionals to report child abuse cases to the appropriate governmental agency.

Following is a case in which a nurse is the one to learn of child abuse and has to decide where her duties lie.

S., a two-year-old, died in a local hospital as the result of falling down a flight of concrete steps. His mother was very withdrawn and had stayed with her son very little. Ms. P. was the nurse on duty when the accident happened, and she thought that child abuse could have been involved, but there way no way it could be proven.

Months later, Ms. P. received a phone call from the boy's mother. The mother was very upset and burst into tears. As Ms. P. tried to calm her, she suddenly confessed that she had pushed her son down the stairs. She said her nerves were bad at that time but with the exception of thinking of her son and what happened, she was better. She said, "Please don't say anything about this."

The mother was divorced and was receiving welfare. She had another small son, a one-year-old, in her care [Carroll and Humphrey, 1979, p. 113].

In most states one's legal duty would be to report the information to appropriate authorities. Our question here is whether it would be *morally* acceptable to break the confidence. Are we showing disrespect for the dignity and autonomy of the client if we fail to keep private the knowledge we have gained of their wrong-doing (child abuse)? By violating another's rights as a person (which child abuse is), have they surrendered their claim to confidentiality? Would they have legitimate grounds of complaint against us if we divulged the knowledge in these types of cases? Is the fact that this mother has another child in her care who is also in great danger of being abused a sufficient basis for breaching the confidence?

We have seen that privacy must be preserved. Personal control over information about oneself and access to that information is essential to being a person. Without such control, human relationships such as love, friendship, and dialogue would be stymied. For these reasons, confidentiality is a *prima facie* duty of the health professional. But do these considerations require us to maintain confidentiality in cases in which doing so is detrimental to the rights and interests of others? Can we convincingly argue that in cases of violation of the rights of others one no longer has a duty to maintain the confidence? Surely we would want to be free to breach confidences in order to protect someone who is endangered, especially a vulnerable child.

A *prima facie* duty to maintain confidences does allow for breaking them when more stringent duties conflict with keeping the confidence. (If it did not, the duty would be an absolute rather than a *prima facie* one.) Hence we must ask: Does the health professional have any other conflicting duties in this situation that are more stringent than the duty to maintain confidentiality?

In some situations, we have a moral duty to protect others from harm, such as when an able-bodied adult sees a child drowning in three feet of water. All he needs to do to save the child is to wade into the water and carry the child out. Similarly, if a health professional were to discover that a child were in imminent danger because of action by his parents (e.g., child abuse, neglect, or inability to care for the child) and the child could be spared if the health professional made a few phone calls, we would feel that the health professional had a *prima facie* duty to do so.

Suppose, however, that making these phone calls would necessarily result in divulging confidential information. The health professional has two conflicting *prima facie* duties: the duty to maintain client confidentiality and the duty to prevent harm. Which duty takes priority?

We cannot argue generally that the duty to prevent harm always takes priority over the duty to maintain confidentiality or vice versa. Too many factors that vary from case to case are involved, such as the degree of harm that could occur, the likelihood of harm actually occurring (most cases are not as clear-cut about this as our hypothetical case), and the means available for preventing the anticipated harm. In each situation, these various factors must be considered. The greater the degree of harm, the greater the likelihood of harm, the greater the chance of preventing the harm with the least amount of disruption of one's own schedule, and so on, the stronger the duty to act. Considering all these factors as well as the factors (discussed earlier) that contribute to the strength of the duty to maintain confidentiality, one must decide which duty has priority.

One additional factor must be considered in the particular situations we have been examining, namely, the fact that the client's action (or inaction) is the cause of another person being in imminent danger. All would agree that a person's autonomy does not extend beyond his or her own person to the person or property of others. We owe confidentiality to another because of our more-basic duty of respecting that person's autonomy. If a person's right to autonomy does not provide a protective cover for harming another, surely the right of confidentiality (which is based on autonomy) cannot provide one with protective cover when harming another. The protection of confidentiality does not extend to those actions which are incompatible with the rights of an innocent third party.

3. Generally speaking, confidentiality may be breached when it is necessary to protect the public from a clear and present danger. Cases frequently cited are of clients with serious medical problems whose occupations make them responsible for the lives of many other persons—for example, an airline pilot with failing eyesight or a bus driver with a serious heart condition. Frequently cited is the highly publicized case in New York City some years ago of a bus driver who had a heart attack and caused his bus to plunge into the East River, killing thirty people. The driver's physician had know about the heart condition and had cautioned him not to drive, but felt he should not report it to the bus company.

We can imagine that, as a good citizen, the doctor would have liked to report the heart condition to ensure that the safety of the bus-riding public not be jeapardized. As a health professional, however, he felt his stronger duty lay with client confidentiality.

Some, in arguing against this physician's position, would claim that he had a *duty* to report his client's heart condition. A utilitarian would appeal to the duty to maximize the general good and point to the disastrous results of failure to report it as sufficient ground for being obligated to break the confidence. The danger of this argument, however, is that it can quickly reduce the individual to an entity to be manipulated for the common good. Autonomy of the individual becomes subordinated to the good of the greater number.

If, on the contrary, we argue that the physician is *permitted* to breach the confidence because his or her duty to prevent harm is in conflict with the duty to maintain confidentiality, and then proceed with an argument concerning the limits of autonomy and privacy vis-à-vis conflicts with others such as we presented above, we do not run the risk of subordinating the individual to the collective. Yet in conformity with our moral intuitions we provide a basis for breaking the confidence.

A necessary additional protection of clients' rights is to make clear at the outset (perhaps by legislation for some types of cases) what the limits of confidentiality are to be. That is, it should generally be understood that if certain kinds of information are gained by health professionals, they are free to divulge that information to relevant authorities or affected parties. (This is a weaker requirement than one that makes it a *duty* to report such information.)

The position that the health professional may breach confidentiality either to right a wrong or to promote good is much more difficult to defend than is the position just presented, which allows us to break confidentiality to *prevent* harm. (See the ordering of these principles in Chapter 1.)

Consider the following case of the confession of a crime.

Many years ago a member of the government was assassinated in the centre of the capital city. Several people were arrested; one of them was injured and he was taken to the hospital. The police were investigating the case. The injured man was examined by the police but in the end it was concluded by them that he was innocent. Nothing was proved to be against him.

However, he showed many signs of anxiety and after some days he called the night nurse. He confessed to her that he was the one who had murdered the member of the government. The nurse assured him that she would not tell anyone about it but she strongly advised him to confess to the priest of the hospital. He eventually did so. Two people now knew the important secret but neither felt they could tell the police about it. Both of them felt they were tied to secrecy by their professional obligation to the patient. The priest visited the patient quite often [Tate, 1977, p. 24].

We will be more likely to agree with the judgment of the nurse (and the priest) that the confidentiality should *not* be breached if we see breaking the confidence either as righting a wrong (removing evil) or as promoting a good, than if we see the case as one of preventing harm. Suppose that the injured man or his cohorts were intent upon attacking other government leaders and would do so if the confidence were not broken. The duty to prevent such harm is more compelling and hence more persuasively supersedes the duty to maintain confidentiality than are a health professional's duties to see to it that a wrong-doer is brought to justice or that some (nonhealth-related) good is advanced (e.g., the rebel forces are dealt a serious blow and the government's power is solidified).

Related to the question of when, if ever, confidentiality may be breached is the question of how confidential records are to be kept. Often the nurse must work with medical records. Computerized health data systems make inadvertent and surreptitious breaches of confidentiality possible on a much wider scale than did earlier record systems. Counter-balancing the gains in efficiency and accuracy are the additional dangers of the individual's lack of control over the information about himself or herself and the potentially greater damage to the client, whose confidentiality is violated by unauthorized access to the computerized records.

Greater care than may have been necessary in the past must be taken to limit access to confidential medical records. Clearly, situations such as the following case demonstrate a complete lack of sensitivity to the issue of access to records in order to protect client confidentiality.

While working in the emergency room, I saw two teenage females who allegedly took a bottle (100 tablets) of aspirin each. They both appeared lethargic, but their vital signs were stable and by the time the physician had seen them, they were alert and able to walk without assistance. They did not exhibit any of the signs of overdose, but the physician did order their stomachs pumped and the lab test showed only a slight amount of aspirin in their stomach contents. They were discharged from the emergency room in the custody of their boyfriends.

The next afternoon the local paper reported this case and I was very upset that the report was written verbatim exactly as I had recorded it on the out-patient record. I had given out no information. I immediately asked whether these records were taken to the medical record department and was assured that they were. My next question was how did this information get in the paper exactly as I had written.

When asked why the editor of the local paper came to the hospital so often, the director of nurses told me that he had been a hospital administrator before taking the editor position. Upon learning this information, I asked if he still had his master key to the hospital, including records, and was told that he did. All the persons in authority knew of this situation but no one tried to see to it that this situation was remedied [Carroll and Humphrey, 1979, pp. 114-15].

If we are going to show any sensitivity to client confidentiality, privacy, and autonomy, we must carefully restrict access. For example, confidential information could be graded according to different levels of sensitivity. Users of the system could be assigned codes that provide them with access only to the particular grades of confidential information to which they must have access. Some such safeguards are morally required.

In addition to the question of access, the moral dimensions of medical record-keeping must include a decision on what is to be done with recorded information that is no longer appropriate. Human beings grow and change and, in important respects, become different persons than they once were. Yet a medical record can have the effect of locking someone into a particular pattern or syndrome in the eyes of health practitioners. Being locked in is to have one's autonomy undercut. This process is understood and explained well by the nurse who provides the following examples of moral problems arising with long-term medical records:

As a school nurse, I am faced with the ethical problem of protection of information about the pupils. Accurate records about the pupils help the nurses maintain good care for pupils over a long period of time. The health records for each student accompany him from kindergarten on through his entire educational experience. If he changes residence and/or schools his record is transferred with him.

The record contains information of the state of his health at regular intervals. It builds a continuous record of his physical and psychological development. It also contains information that pertains to family life and environmental factors, which may influence his health and be pertinent in giving health care. The rationale for keeping this complete a record is clearly for the student's benefit. It provides for continuity and follow-up in care and treatment; it records successive treatments and observations for evaluation of progress; it passes on needed information to health personnel when there is a change in the individuals responsible for the student's health.

The ethical problem occurs when particular accounts, which once seemed essential for helping the student, remain in the record over a long period of years. The record may leave a mark that will accompany the student for many years. It might well change the attitude of someone toward him and even insult or injure him in his later relationships. Medical records should not be able to leave such a mark on a child.

Some examples of problems from records:

A boy sent to the mental health clinic because of many adolescent problems. Because of this note in his record, he was not accepted in the army with those from his particular age group. Many discussions ensued and at a later time he was allowed to serve as a regular soldier and had no difficulty in fulfilling his responsibilities.

A 6-year old girl hospitalized after her father attempted to have intercourse with her. Her father was later hospitalized. The details of this episode which were essential to her care at the time remained in her record in the schools and accompanied her for many years. The mother of this pupil is a prostitute. The pupil has a brother and a sister both of whom have unknown fathers.

It is possible in all these instances that the mental trauma to the child will cause a problem in the future. The information might be of use in treating later illnesses. However, the initial treatment may have alleviated the problem for all time and his development will continue normally. Questions asked by later health personnel with access to these records might be the only way that these incidents would later disturb an otherwise normal adjustment to life [Tate, 1977, pp. 22–23].

Because the facts of each case vary so greatly, we cannot set out any straight-forward guidelines for deciding when information should be kept in the record and when it should be removed. The decision in particular cases requires the expertise of various health professionals. But it is not simply a medical question; it is a question as well of client autonomy. Surely no one is better qualified to speak to that issue than the competent client himself or herself. Hence, there should be periodic opportunities for the client to review (with the guidance of appropriate health professionals) her or his own confidential medical record so that the client can know if items in the record are affecting the care she or he receives and the perception health professionals have of her or him.

We have seen that the fundamental moral reason for the confidentiality of medical records is that it protects the client's privacy and autonomy. When the principle of confidentiality of medical records is appealed to in order to limit the client's access to his or her own records, this is a perversion of the principle. In special cases there may be good (paternalistic) reasons not to allow a client access to his or her records. But the principle of confidentiality is not available as a ground for limiting the client's own access.

Conclusion

Taking as our starting point the Kantian principle of respect for persons and the ranking of the duties to refrain from harming another, to prevent harm, to remove evil, and to promote good laid down in Chapter 1, we have examined four primary duties of health professionals: the duty to obtain informed consent, the duty to refrain from coercion, the duty to tell the truth, and the duty to maintain confidentiality. We have shown how these duties are derived from the basic principles set forth in the first chapter. We have also examined precisely how these duties are to be applied in actual cases. Regarding conflict of duty situations, we have offered guidance for determining which duties should be given priority. Since making moral decisions is a complex process that requires each person to think for himself or herself, no simple formulas or recipes can be provided, nor would the thoughtful person want them. Instead, the chapter was designed to help clarify issues and to give reasons for taking one position as opposed to another.

Were the nurse not also a member of a larger community, our discussion could be concluded at this point. We have examined the major moral issues facing the nurse at the client's bedside. But, of course, the nurse does not live in a vacuum. The nurse is a member of a profession and a community. The individual perspective of the bedside nurse must be augmented by the social perspective of the nurse as member of the profession, as employee, and as responsible citizen. The next three chapters address issues of nurses' collective responsibilities.

6

The Nurse as a Member of a Profession

Members of the nursing profession for a variety or reasons, including the nature of the profession but also economic exploitation and sexism (see Ashley, 1977), have been "caught in the middle." On the one hand, for example, the nurse is hired to carry out the directives of the physician and to support the policy of the hospital administration. The system cannot function as presently constituted without such cooperation and support to carrying out the decisions and policies of those higher up in the hierarchy. Yet, on the other hand, the nurse is legally and morally accountable for her or his judgments exercised and actions taken. "Neither physician's prescriptions nor the employing agency's policies relieve the nurse of ethical or legal accountability for actions taken and judgments made" (ANA, 1976, p. 10).

A common predicament of nurses is expressed in the April issue of *Nursing '78* by a nurse at a West Coast university hospital. She says:

Our biggest problem right now is that our nursing leadership at the administrative level is completely impotent. They have no voting rights on any committee that has direct control over the hospital and/or nursing. Worse, the acting director and her associate have no idea of taking any power into their own hands, where it rightfully belongs. They ask permission to improve staffing ratios, by increasing or closing beds, and when they're turned down, say to us "Sorry girls! Work doubles" [Godfrey, 1978, pp. 101-2].

The overwork and understaffing not only make working conditions less than desirable for the nurse, they clearly endanger clients. When, for example, one registered nurse and an aide must try to care for 30 to 36 clients who have just undergone surgery, the situation is very dangerous and health care cannot be delivered in accordance with acceptable standards.

We can all sympathize with the nurse who wrote the following:

I am supposed to be responsible for the control and safety of techniques used in the operating theatre. I have spent many hours teaching the technicians and the aides the routines necessary for maintaining aseptic conditions during surgery. They have learned to prepare materials and to maintain an adequate supply for all needs. They have learned to handle supplies with good technique.

I find it is extremely difficult to have these appropriate routines carried out constantly by employees with little theoretical background or understanding. The surgeons are frequently breaking techniques and respond in a belligerent manner when breaks in technique are broght to their attention. I find a reminder of techniques often brings a determined response to ignore the remainder and proceed with surgery. For a male surgeon to be questioned by a female nurse is a serious breach of respect to them.

One day a surgeon wore the same gown for two successive operations even though there were other gowns available. I quietly called this to his attention, but I had no authority which really allowed me to control his behavior for the good of the patient. In this situation even the hospital administrator was of no help to me [Tate, 1977, pp. 47-48].

This nurse is responsible for the control and safety of techniques used in the operating rooms. The conditions over which she is responsible have fallen below acceptable standards. Although she has done her best, the assigned task has not been accomplished. The clients who have a right to expect, and have paid for, a safe and aseptic operating room have been let down.

Nursing is the largest group of health care professionals within the vast health care delivery system—a system that, despite some dramatic achievements, is increasingly under attack as dehumanizing, exploitative, and cost-ineffective. Despite the seeming powerlessness of an individual nurse, taken collectively nursing, more than any other health care profession, is a necessary component in the delivery of health care. The present system could not have developed without nursing. If all nurses were to walk out tomorrow, the system would collapse. This cannot be said for any other group of health care professionals, including physicians. Hence, if the delivery of health care is substandard (as I believe it is), the nurse is not merely a victim of the system (along with the rest of us), but she or he is also an accomplice. As an accomplice she or he shares responsibility for the system's deficiencies. The nurse's plight is by no means unique. The paradoxical plight of the nurse who is both powerless and powerful, responsible yet not responsible, is a plight in which we almost all find ourselves in some aspects of our lives.

One way to try to make sense of these paradoxical situations—to be explored in this chapter—is to introduce the notion of collective responsibility. Two dramatic and widely discussed illustrations are the prosecution's case against certain middle-level Nazis after World War II and the defense's case for First Lieutenant William Calley, charged with murder at MyLai in southeast Asia.

In the prosecution case, blame for the actions of certain individual members of the collective is ascribed to all members. Karl Jaspers expressed this view when he said: "Every German is made to share the blame for the crimes committed in the name of the Reich . . . inasmuch as we let such a regime arise among us" (Quoted in Cooper, 1972, p. 86). In condemning every German, Jaspers is not merely blaming each German for his active or passive tolerance of the Nazis; he is saying that "the world of German ideas," "German thought," and "national tradition" are to blame. Collective responsibility is used as a net from which no member of the collective can escape.

In the defense case, the individual whose behavior has fallen below the acceptable standard is shielded from the full weight of blame, because the weight is shifted to the collective. It is the collective, the system, that must bear the brunt of the burden, rather than the individual. In the Calley case it was claimed that Americans as a group failed to perform as they could have been expected to.

In a recent survey of nurses' attitudes (Godfrey, 1978, Part II, p. 110), this defense strategy was tacitly used. It was reported that, although nurses saw themselves as performing well given the work conditions, they "felt they ought somehow to deliver even when the system won't let them." The writers of the report indicate that this blame is misplaced ("not deserved"). Although performing below the acceptable standard, the nurses were not to be blamed because as individuals each was doing the best possible for him or her in the situation. The system itself was to be blamed.

If the blame appropriately ascribed in a situation is no greater than the sum of all the ascriptions of blame to the individuals, we do not have a case of collective responsibility except in a weak (distributive) sense. By collective responsibility in the strong (nondistributive) sense, as the term is to be used here, we mean that the responsibility of the group is not equivalent to that of the individuals; that is, the whole is not equal to the sum of its parts.

It is incontrovertible that we do ascribe responsibility to collectives in this strong sense. To use an example of D. E. Cooper's, if we say that the local tennis club is responsible for its closure, we do not necessarily or usually mean that the officers of the club or any particular members are responsible for its closure. The blame cannot be attributed to any particular individual or to the officers of the club, since no person failed to do what was expected of him. Yet something was missing. "It was just a bad club as a whole." From the claim that the local tennis club is responsible for its closure, no statements about particular individuals follow. "This is so," as Cooper says, "because the existence of a collective is compatible with a varying membership. No determinate set of individuals is necessary for the existence of a collective" (Cooper, 1968, pp. 260–62).

As R. S. Downie has argued, "To provide an adequate description of the actions, purposes, and responsibilities of a certain range of collectives, such as governments, armies, colleges, incorporated business firms, etc., we must make use of concepts which logically cannot be analyzed in individualistic terms" (Downie, 1972, p. 69).

The question to ask then is what set of conditions must obtain in order properly to ascribe nondistributive collective blame or responsibility. The conditions advanced by Cooper in his article "Responsibility and the 'System' " (1972, pp. 90–91) are sufficiently accurate and refined for purposes of this book. These conditions are:

1. Members of a group perform undesirable acts.

2. Their performing these acts is partly explained by their acting in accordance with the "way of life" of the group (i.e. the rules, mores, customs, etc. of the group).

3. These characteristics of the group's "way of life" are below the standards we might reasonably expect the group to meet.

4. It is not necessarily the case that members of the group, in performing the acts, are falling below standards we can reasonably expect individuals to meet.

A few comments about these conditions are in order. Clearly, we do not *hold* an individual or a group responsible—that is, following its etymology: having liability to answer to a *charge*—if undesirable acts have not been performed. When no undesirable acts occur, the question of blame or responsibility in the sense of liability does not arise. Hence the need for condition 1.

The second condition is not strictly necessary. It does seem, as Virginia Held has argued (1970), that when special conditions obtain even a random collection of individuals can be held responsible (a claim denied by condition 2). Nonetheless, for present purposes— consideration of collective responsibility of members of a profession— this stronger claim need not be defended. The most-plausible cases for ascribing collective responsibility are those cases in which the group has distinctive characteristics, has a sense of solidarity and cohesion (for example, feels "vicarious pride and shame" [Feinberg, 1968, p. 677]) and members identify themselves as members of the group (for example, "Who are you?" "I am a nurse"), and some of these group feelings or characteristics are appealed to in explaining the acts in question. An illustration: If the citizens of Syldavia can be characterized as being rather hostile and distrustful of foreigners, and their customs, laws, and policies reflect this, then when some border guards—overzealously carrying out the Syldavian policy—kill some visiting dignitaries, we blame not only the border guards but the Syldavians. In contrast, if these border guards steal from the visiting dignitaries, in accounting for this behavior we would not be inclined to appeal to any larger group feelings or characteristics, and we definitely would not wish to ascribe collective blame.

We have seen in the variety of cases discussed above that it is when a collective fails to live up to what can reasonably be expected of it—i.e., it falls below an acceptable standard—that it can incur collective blame. Hence the need for condition 3.

Condition 4 is necessary because the standards applied to groups may be different from those applied to individuals. For example, we may feel that the nurse (in the case cited above) who was charged with responsibility for the control and safety of techniques used in the operating rooms adequately met her obligations. She did not fall below standards we can reasonably expect an individual to meet. After all, as Joel Feinberg has argued, "No individual person can be blamed for not being a hero or a saint." Yet, as Feinberg goes on to say, "A whole people can be blamed for not producing a hero when the times require it, especially when the failure can be charged to some discernible element in the group's 'way of life' that militates against heroism" (Feinberg, 1968, p. 687). Although Feinberg was not referring to this case or to the collective responsibility of the nursing profession (he was talking about a Jesse James train robbery case), his remarks are especially apt for this case and in many other situations within the nursing profession.

One can readily see that conditions outlined for properly ascribing nondistributive collective responsibility obtain in many situations within professions. Professions more than most other collectives are bound together by common aspirations, values, methodologies, and training. In too many cases, they also have similar socio-economic backgrounds and are of the same sex and ethnic group. As we have seen, the more cohesive the group, the less problematic the ascription of collective responsibility. The fact that professions such as nursing promulgate codes of ethics or standards of behavior, toward which they expect members to strive, provides a clear criterion for judging whether the actual practices of the profession fall below standards to which we can reasonably hold the group.

In addition to meeting these formal criteria for ascribing collective responsibility, there are several other reasons unique to the professions for ascribing collective responsibility in certain situations.

A. There are several ways by which one becomes responsible. One can be *saddled* with it by circumstances, one can have responsibility *assigned* to one, or one can deliberately *assume* responsibility (Baier, 1972, p. 52). Typically a profession is chosen. In choosing the profession, one *assumes* the responsibility concomitant with being a professional. One chooses to adopt the values, methodology, and "way of life" of the profession. Such choice is much less prominent with most other basic group affiliations. One does not choose family membership, region of birth, usually not citizenship, and often not military service. Once in the profession, of course, as one goes about his or her job he or she will also sometimes be saddled with responsibility by circumstances and be assigned responsibility. But these assignments are all within the context of choice: to assume professional responsibility provides the backdrop for all his or her professional activities. Hence, as a professional, more than most other group affiliations, one sees oneself as a member of the group and has—with eyes open—chosen the identification.

B. Nurses (as is, of course, also the case in several other professions) have been vested by the state with the power to regulate and control nursing practice. This collective power or right—given exclusively to the profession—has a concomitant collective responsibility to see to it that acceptable standards are maintained. Since it is possible that each individual nurse, including officers of the American Nursing Association, is meeting acceptable standards in her or his own assignments and yet the group's "way of life" must be characterized as below an acceptable standard, appeal to collective responsibility is one of the tools the public has at its disposal to try to ensure adequate nursing and general health care. Obviously in these cases (when no individual has failed to meet her or his legal obligation), the public does not have recourse to law suits against individuals.

C. Supposedly as a means to protect the public, the licensing statutes of the states allow only those who have passed certain state requirements to practice nursing. One result of this is that the profession, which is by law also self-regulatory, becomes a protected monopoly. If a person is going to receive nursing care, this care must be provided by a member of the profession. If nursing care is to be upgraded, it must be from within with, at most, prodding from without. Quite clearly, one of the most-effective tools for such prodding is that of demonstrating collective responsibility, a responsibility that goes beyond the sum of each individual's responsibility.

From the discussion thus far, it is evident that the appeal to collective responsibility when some substandard behavior or undesirable act has occurred is a two-edged sword. It can be used to show that, despite undesirable performances or actions or conditions within a collective, a particular member of the collective is not individually responsible. But it can also be used to show that, despite the fact that the behavior of individuals does not fall below standards we can reasonably require individuals to meet (given that we cannot *demand* that an individual be a hero), the group's conduct is below the standards we can reasonably expect the group to meet. One of the reasons the weapon of collective responsibility looks suspect in the widely discussed World War II prosecution and Vietnam conflict defense cases is that only one edge of the sword is used, while the other edge is conveniently ignored.

If conditions for properly ascribing collective responsibility are satisfied, to the extent that the individual is exonerated, the group is indicted. To the degree the individual *qua* individual is indicted, the group is exonerated. Either way the individual group member bears responsibility. For any member of a collective but especially (for reasons cited above) for a professional, it is not enough to know that one has done all that could be expected of him or her as an individual. The arm of responsibility for a professional has a longer reach than that of the individual.

Specific situations within the nursing profession illustrate the two edges of the sword of collective responsibility. These situations should be seen within the context of the rapid evolution of the nursing profession. In recent years there has been considerable effort both within and outside the profession (e.g., the medical profession) to upgrade the requirements for licensure. These efforts have borne results. The scope of the professional nurse has expanded greatly, as exemplified by medical assistant programs and their use by medical doctors in certain areas. The history of the struggle first to adopt a code of ethics for American nurses and then to revise it reflects this evolution. Tentative codes were presented in the 1920s, 1930s, and 1940s. These efforts were met by opposition from those who feared the professionalization of nursing. A striking instance of this is the advice given by a physician to one of the earliest advocates of a code of ethics for American nurses: "Be good women but do not have a code of ethics" (Dock, 1912, p. 129). Not until 1950 was a code of ethics adopted.

The code has been changed several times since then, the most recent being in 1976. Two of the most-interesting changes from our vantage point have been the following: early versions of the code stated that the nurse had an obligation to carry out the physician's orders. As we saw in Chapter 1, the 1968 and 1976 versions of the code instead stress the nurse's obligation to the client. The physician just mentioned who advised against having a code may have foreseen this development! Whereas earlier versions of the code pointed to an obligation to sustain confidence in associates, in the revised codes the nurse's obligation is to protect the client from incompetent, unethical, or illegal practice from any quarter. (See Sward, 1978, for a discussion of these and other changes in the versions of the code.)

With this background, it is apparent why nursing is an especially interesting example of collective responsibility in the professions. The fundamental issue in the ongoing struggle to upgrade the profession—reflected in the code changes—has been that of accountability, the willingness to make decisions and to accept responsibility for these decisions. The crucial question in the attempt to upgrade the profession is that of the interface of individual and collective responsibility.

The author of an article in the *Quarterly Record of the Massachusetts General Hospital Nurses Alumnae Association* wrote about "blame avoidance" behavior in nurses. As explained, blame avoidance behavior is exhibited when the nurse says such things as "I did this because the supervisor told me to do it," or "the doctor ordered it," or "the hospital rules demanded it." The author maintains that accountability requires that the nurse can say, "I did this because in my best judgment it is what the patient needed" (quoted in Durand, 1978, p. 19). Setting aside the many good qualities common to nurses, blame avoidance behavior does seem to be one of the more-prevalent, endemic faults of the nursing profession. As we have seen, a concerted effort by many within the profession has made inroads on this "way of life" of the profession.

These efforts have been made without explicit appeal to the concept of collective responsibility. As a result, judgment in cases of blame avoidance and other unacceptable or undesirable behavior has tended to be either too lenient or too harsh. That is, either (a) one judges that the individual nurse caught in the middle and in difficult circumstances has done all one can reasonably expect her or him to do. After all, we cannot expect or demand that she or he be a hero or a saint. Hence, the nurse is exonerated, but the unacceptable practice or conditon continues unabated. Or (b) one focuses on professional responsibility and the fact that, if some individuals do not stand up against substandard practices—no matter what the odds of thereby improving the situation and no matter at what price to the individual—

these practices likely will not be stopped. If the nurse does not take the action that would probably cost her her position, but that would ensure the best care possible for clients in her care, the nurse is judged to be a moral coward.

For example, in the case of the nurse charged with responsibility for maintaining a safe and aseptic operating room, without appeal to the concept of collective responsibility we are likely to say one of the following: (1) She has done all we can require of her (she has asked the surgeon to comply; she does not have the authority or status to demand compliance to proper procedures; the lack of compliance quite properly was followed by a report to the hospital administration.) Or (2) she has not done all we can require of her (she cannot allow dangerous violations of operating room aseptic standards to take place; in doing so, she is failing to carry out her assignment and is allowing the client's life to be placed in jeopardy; she should not be cowed by the surgeon's arrogance and sexism; even at the risk of losing her job, she cannot allow the operation to take place in these conditions).

The problem is that (1) is too lenient a judgment and (2) is too harsh. We cannot require the nurse *qua* individual to do more than she has done. But the nurse *qua* nurse shares blame with her colleagues in such cases, despite the much greater blame that must be placed on the surgeon who violates reasonable requirements. The lack of aggressive advocacy for the client's welfare and the willingness to be dominated by the (usually male) physician or surgeon (unfortunate if understandable "ways of life" of the nursing profession), which partially explain this nurse's behavior, are below the standard we can rightfully expect the group authorized to provide nursing services to meet. Appeal to collective responsibility yields a judgment neither too harsh nor too lenient.

This judgment conforms to the moral intuitions of the nurses surveyed who were mentioned earlier. Despite a feeling that as individuals they were doing all that could reasonably be required of them in their circumstances, they still felt dissatisfied with their performance. As nurses they felt blame for falling short of the mark set for the profession.

This dissatisfaction, when seen in the light of collective responsibility, can be turned to positive use. The nurse who has done all that is required of him or her as an individual need not suffer debilitating guilt. Guilt, in such cases, is misplaced; her or his individual actions do not warrant guilt. And, in contrast to nondistributive collective responsibility, there is no nondistributive collective guilt. "Guilt," as Feinberg has said, "consists in the intentional transgression of a prohibition . . . There can be no such thing as vicarious guilt" (Feinberg, 1968, p. 676). Nevertheless, although rightfully free of guilt, she or he cannot be complacent. She or he is a member of a group that stands judged (i.e., is liable) and must, with her or his colleagues, take appropriate steps to alleviate the undesirable conditions. It is not enough for a professional to do all that is required of her or him as an individual. Having freely accepted the privileges and benefits of the profession, one's responsibility in the areas of professional competence is greater than would be that of an equally skilled and knowledgeable individual who was not a member of the profession.

In order to meet this larger responsibility, as the American Nursing Association has recognized, "there should be an established mechanism for the reporting and handling of incompetent, unethical, or illegal practice within the employment setting so that such reporting can go through official channels and be done without fear of reprisal. The nurse should be knowledgeable about the mechanism and be prepared to utilize it if necessary" (Sward, 1978, p. 8).

Paradoxically, if such machinery which collective responsibility requires were put in place, individual accountability would increase and the need to appeal to collective responsibility would decrease. If reporting incompetent, unethical, or illegal conduct could be done effectively through official channels and without fear of reprisal, such reporting—which under more-dangerous and less-effective circumstances is not required—would be morally required of the individual. Hence, it may be that a profession should strive to organize itself and regulate itself to such a degree that the conditions for proper ascription of collective responsibility do not arise. But this is not the situation within the nursing profession at the present. Therefore, the notion of collective responsibility is a timely weapon of considerable force for those who are working toward upgrading the nursing profession and the delivery of health care.

7

The Nurse as an Employee

Of all the moral issues facing the nurse as an employee, none is more difficult and divisive than deciding whether to go on strike, the issue we shall explore in this chapter. Its difficulty as a moral dilemma arises from the fact that compelling moral reasons can be given in support of both sides of the question.

A nurse is quoted in a recent article in the *New York Times* (March 25, 1980) as saying that when nurses strike, "they talk about better patient care, but the bottom line is 'How much are you going to give me?'" Since bill collectors are as persistent with nurses as with professors, plumbers, and police officers, it is hardly surprising if, for most individual nurses on strike, wages are of greater and more compelling concern than demands for improved client care. Yet it would be a mistake to conclude from this that the expressions of concern about quality client care are no more than smoke screens. Nurses as professionals have and take seriously the collective responsibility of maintaining and improving the quality of nursing care. The question to be discussed is whether (and if so, when) the strike is a morally acceptable weapon for nurses to use in attempting to maintain and improve the conditions necessary for proper nursing practice and their self-respect.

Too often, discussions of the moral duties of health professionals give the impression that the list of duties is exhausted when one has gone through those which pertain to the health professional as individual practitioner: the duty to respect a client's autonomy, the duty to obtain informed consent, the duty to maintain confidentiality, the duty to safeguard privacy. But health professionals do not work in a vacuum. Because of society's interest in their activity, their practice is regulated by the state. Specifically, as mentioned in the previous chapter, the nursing profession is given the legal status of a protected monopoly (no one may practice nursing unless licensed by the profession) and the authority to control its own practice. In exchange, society asks the profession to deliver high-quality nursing services. By accepting the role of nurse, one—along with one's colleagues— assumes responsibility (1) for maintaining and improving standards of nursing, (2) for maintaining conditions of employment conducive to high-quality nursing care, (3) for contributing to the development and implementation of community and national health needs, and (4) for making the most-efficient and -effective use of nursing resources.

To exercise these duties, it is necessary for nurses to act in concert— for example, to work through professional associations or unions or to form independent groups within one's employment setting. If these collective efforts meet resistance or prove ineffectual, it may be difficult or impossible to fulfill these duties without taking further action, such as engaging in a strike or work slowdown. Yet such action may come into conflict with a variety of the nurses' other duties, including their collective duty to provide nursing care to all in need of it and their duties as practitioners to specific clients currently under their care. This potential for conflicts of duty is what makes the question of the nurses' right to strike a morally difficult and complex one.

The issue is compelling because many nurses find themselves in situations in which it is next to impossible to fulfill their collective responsibilities. Frequently (as we discussed in several previous chapters) nurses lack power relative to administrators and other health professionals, such as doctors. Their proper place is often seen as being "at the physician's side"—a position of low esteem. Nurse supervisors often have neither the ability nor the desire forcefully to defend members of their staff in disputes with other health professionals or administrators. Far too often nurses are assigned too many clients or ordered to do tasks that lie outside the range of their training or expertise. These and many other factors militate against high-quality nursing care.

We have already seen some of the causes of nurses' relative powerlessness and low esteem. Among the most important ones are the following:

1. The pervasive sexism of our culture. Sexist attitudes appear to have shaped society's expectations that nurses will perform the stereotypical female helping role. These same attitudes are reflected in (some) nurses' images of themselves as handmaidens of the physician or as surrogate mothers.

2. The class background of nurses. Whereas over the years most nurses have come from the lower half of the socio-economic spectrum, typically physicians have come from classes in the upper half.

3. Their relative lack of education. Many nurses lack a quality liberal arts education—a factor that sets them apart from most other professional groups. And their medical training is no match for that of doctors.

4. Their relatively low pay. This may be a consequence of the causes cited above, yet it in turn contributes to the low esteem accorded nurses. In our society esteem is, at least loosely, correlated with level of income. (The average nurse's salary in the United States is around $13,000–$14,000—considerably less than the pay of doctors and other professionals.)

High-quality nursing care is unlikely to be widely available if nurses' positions of relative powerlessness and low esteem persist. Only if the conditions just cited are ameliorated is there a possibility of change— change that is essential if nurses are to fulfill the collective duties outlined above. Of course, to change these conditions is no easy task. Yet there is a growing awareness that things can and should be different. Through sheer dint of numbers (there are more nurses than any other health professionals) and because of the importance of nursing services, the *potential* for power to make these changes is undeniable.

In a variety of ways, these offending conditions and attitudes are being challenged. Two examples follow: New models of the nurse's role, such as the one discussed in Chapter 2, have stressed independent, professional judgment and action primarily on behalf of the client, as opposed to being primarily an extension of the physician. These models emphasize the distinctive contribution of nursing (e.g., *caring* for the sick as opposed to physicians' contributions of diagnosing disease and attempting cures). Discussion and adoption of these models help somewhat to overcome the negative effects of the traditional, weak model. A second example (also discussed in Chapter 2) is the American Nursing Association's diligent (and controversial) efforts to upgrade nursing education. The Association has been concerned that nurses' education be adequate to meet the challenges of high-quality nursing in today's world: care that requires skill in handling increasingly complex and sophisticated equipment, advanced training in nursing specialties and subspecialties, and the expertise to take on the lion's share of health education as our society places increasing emphasis on preventive care.

These are just two of any number of ways the nursing profession must work to satisfy its collective responsibility to provide quality nursing care. We turn now to the question of the appropriateness of a possible third way, collective action through strikes. Is the strike one of the paths nurses may follow in attempting to meet their collective responsibilities?

The strike is a technique usually used by labor organizations to exact economic concessions from management. It would be very unusual for a strike not to be premised in large part on demands for better pay and benefits. If such "self-serving" goals are incompatible with exercising professional responsibility, surely a strike by nurses could not be condoned. However, far from being incompatible with professional responsibility, the demand for better wages (we shall argue) is a requirement of professional responsibility.

An increase in compensation must go hand in hand with up-grading of the profession. Just as low pay is correlated with low esteem and low status, low status is linked to the lack of quality nursing care. Low status is a nearly insurmountable impediment to quality care. The economic issue is *not* detachable from the quality-of-care issue. The quest for higher wages as well as better working conditions is part and parcel of the struggle to fulfill the collective responsibilities of the profession.

It may be objected, however, that this line of reasoning blurs an important, traditional distinction between the professional and the laborer or worker. The worker does his or her job for pay, in part because the required tasks lack intrinsic worth. A professional's motives, it has often been argued, should be different. A professional is committed to his or her profession for its own sake and for the sake of those who are its recipients and beneficiaries. Therefore, the argument continues, a professional must refrain from using the strike weapon.

Is this argument persuasive? Its persuasiveness depends on our being able to detach the economic issues from the quality-of-care issues. We have argued, to the contrary, that they are not detachable. Let us consider this issue further. It would appear to be an empirical fact that we are unlikely to get quality people to enter a profession with poor working conditions, low esteem, and low pay. Even if we were to succeed in attracting highly qualified and highly motivated people, it is unlikely that their enthusiasm and morale could be sustained over the years. High drop-out rates, cynicism, and discouragement—all of which presently obtain in nursing—would have to be expected. If all professionals were motivated solely by love of their art and service to humanity, as proponents of the view under challenge wistfully imagine, a strike would indeed be incompatible with professional standing. But since professionals are humans of complex motivation, the image of the professional on which the argument rests is unrealistic.

Since other professional groups (e.g., teachers, interns, and residents) now engage in strike action and appear not to have lost their professional standing, attempts to show that striking is incompatible with professionalism are unlikely to be effective. If we are to find that striking is incompatible with the professional duties of a *nurse*, the conflict will arise from specific nursing duties rather than from general professional obligations.

Before we turn to these specific duties of the nurse, it will be helpful to look more closely at one's activities when striking. To strike is to take collective action, including the refusal to work, with the aim of extracting concessions from one's employer. The refusal to work imposes inconvenience and possibly hardship on those in need of one's services. In the case of strikes by employees such as nurses, the detrimental effect of the strike on the public (those in need of nursing care) is often more immediate and more grave than on the employer. The public's inconvenience is the means by which pressure is put on the employer to come to a settlement agreeable to the striking employees. Were the public in no way inconvenienced, the strike would likely be ineffectual.

Consider the conflict that appears to arise for the striking nurse, given that the means for achieving admittedly worthy goals is the inconvenience and perhaps even the hardship of clients. The modern nurse who functions in accordance with the client advocate model developed in Chapter 2 is committed to working for the client, in that she or he has the special task of caring for the client as a person, of humanizing an otherwise impersonal and sometimes demeaning health care system. Of all health professionals, the nurse is uniquely situated so as to be the most-effective guardian of the client's interests and rights. Perhaps, then, it is this special role of the nurse that makes it wrong for nurses to strike. For a client advocate to be willing to sacrifice a particular client's interests, in order to achieve higher salaries for oneself and one's colleagues, or better care for future clients, at least appears to be contradictory and wrong.

One way out of this seeming impasse is to reject the special role of client advocate. But this is too heavy a price to pay. It would undermine the image and model of nursing that we have found is superior from the moral point of view and is one with which more and more responsible nurses are identifying themselves.

If—contrary to usual circumstances (as we have discussed)—a nurses' strike were *solely* for higher wages (if no quality-of-care issues were on the table and the situation happened to be such that the salary issue were unlikely to affect quality of care because the pay scale were already relatively high), we can see that a strike would be incompatible with the nurses' role as client advocate. Clients are being used as means for advancing nurses' interests. Clients' interests (which the nurse had pledged to advance) are being held hostage. What makes matters most difficult is that the especially stringent duty not to treat clients in this way is not counter-balanced by any other compelling moral duty. The moral duty of the nurse to her or his clients stands in conflict with self-interest—which, of course, does not provide one with a moral basis for failing to do one's moral duty.

On the other hand, if the strike were undertaken with an aim of advancing client care, the case would be quite different. We have the makings of a classic conflict-of-duty situation. The on-going, collective duty to maintain and improve the quality of nursing care appears to be in conflict with specific duties to one's current clients and the collective duty to provide nursing care to the public. When all of these duties cannot be fulfilled, one has to decide which duty ought to take priority over the others.

For those nurses who find themselves in work contexts in which wages, standards, and practice are deficient, our earlier discussion has made clear that concerted action to correct these conditions is obligatory. As is well known, the recent experience of many nursing groups within specific health care facilities is that the only effective way to affect the needed changes is strike action. If, as a matter of fact, a strike is the most-effective, or indeed the only effective, way in a particular situation to make the changes necessary for quality nursing care, the collective responsibilities of nurses require them to strike—*unless* there are other, more-stringent duties (to be considered below)which are binding on them and which would be violated were they to engage in a strike.

An initially appealing yet (as we shall see) unacceptable argument for giving priority to the duty to maintain and improve the quality of care (and, hence, to strike) is the following: the sacrifice of clients' interests resultant from a strike is for the improvement of future nursing care. That is, the sacrifice required of clients is for the good of clients. It would be short-sighted not to see that this is a reasonable price for clients to pay in order to have better care available in the future. Therefore, as in many other areas of our lives, it is reasonable to sacrifice the short-term interests for the long-term ones. Hence, clients cannot reasonably object to a strike under these conditions.

This argument would have some force if the *same* clients whose present interests and needs are sacrificed were the ones to benefit from the future gains. It is one thing to make X sacrifice now for X's (his or her own) later benefit. It is quite another to make X sacrifice now for Y's (another's) later benefit. But in most strikes, the sacrifice required now is for the benefit of others later. It is the yet-unknown client of the future, rather than the present client, whose welfare a strike can advance. The weakness of the argument is that it fails to consider the crucial question of justice (fair treatment of individuals to whom one already has obligations) and simply considers that of over-all consequences.

In an article discussing the morality of strikes by interns and residents, David Bleich asks:

May a person on the way to a class on first-aid instruction ignore the plight of a dying man, on the plea that he must perfect skills which may enable him to rescue a greater number of persons at some future time? . . . No person may plead that an activity designed to advance future societal benefits is justification for ignoring an immediate responsibility. . . . The "here and now" test is a general rule of thumb which may be applied to most situations requiring an ordering of priorities [Bleich and Veatch, 1975, p. 9].

No doubt we can all agree that the person failing to give aid on his way to first-aid instruction stands defenseless. Bleich suggests that this action violates a general principle to the effect that commitment to a course of action designed to increase future good is not a weighty enough reason to exempt one from immediate duties. Were we to apply this principle to the issue at hand in the manner Bleich proposes, we would conclude that a nurse going on strike even for the highest of motives, namely, to benefit future clients, is in the wrong, for she or he is violating immediate responsibilities to clients in need of nursing by inappropriately appealing to future benefits.

Such a conclusion need not be drawn even if we were to accept Bleich's argument. The sort of nurses' strike that would be analogous to his case of the man on his way to a first-aid class would be a case of nurses on strike to improve emergency nursing care and who refuse to respond to an emergency. In order to improve conditions so that more lives can be saved later, a life is lost here and now. Such a strike could not be morally justified—a fact that is generally recognized and honored by striking nurses, who see to it that nursing care in emergency rooms and intensive care units is not withdrawn. Bleich's example is useful in making it clear why withdrawal of services necessary for the maintenance of life cannot be justified.

The central moral question concerning nurses' strikes, however, is whether the withdrawal of nonemergency and nonlifesaving nursing services can be shown to be an acceptable means to the end of better nursing care for future clients. Bleich's general principle cited above (that one may not plead that one's attempt to advance future good exempts one from any immediate responsibility) prohibits withdrawal of these nursing services as well *if* doing so entails ignoring any immediate duties to clients.

Is Bleich's principle one we should accept? Whether or not we accept it will depend on how important we take considerations of consequences to be. We can imagine any number of cases in which greater overall good would be served if we were free to fail to meet an immediate conflicting responsibility. For example, suppose one were ready to proceed with a research project which, if successful, would probably provide us with the means to save numerous lives in the future. It has been determined that the only way the project can go forward is to select subjects from whom truly informed consent is not possible (for whatever reason). Most people would agree that, at least in general, one's immediate duty to his or her research subjects is to obtain genuine informed consent. Most would also agree that this is a very stringent requirement (as we have argued). Yet if the risk to the research subjects were truly minimal and the potential for gain for those benefiting from the research were immense, we may feel that it is appropriate at least to consider whether an appeal to future societal benefits is sufficient to outweigh this immediate and serious responsibility. If we feel such a consideration is appropriate, our position entails a rejection of Bleich's principle. On the other hand, we may feel consideration of consequences is illegitimate here.

In deciding for or against Bleich's principle, the crux of the matter is how weighty we consider the duty to work for future societal benefits to be. The ethical principles set forth in Chapter 1 allow for a middle position between that of the strict Kantian, who would see a consideration of consequences as illegitimate, and the utilitarian, who would see it as the only factor to be considered. We took the Kantian respect for persons principle and the principle of beneficence as basic. On this modified Kantian view, it is not wrong to consider consequences; however, in doing so one may not run roughshod over another's autonomy or fail to respect others as persons. The fundamental question that one must ask concerning this case is whether the proper balance has been struck between the duty to respect the research subjects as persons while carrying out one's duty of beneficence, which is the role of a research scientist.

We have established that nurses have a clear and compelling duty to see to it that future nursing care will be better than the substandard care available in certain facilities and locales. Contrary to Bleich, it is too stringent to declare *a priori* that all other immediate duties must take priority in conflict-of-duty situations. What must be determined is whether the duty to work toward better nursing care in the future should, in the particular situation at issue, take precedence over any other duty with which it conflicts.

In place of Bleich's principle, let us adopt the following procedural rule: all the various duties of nurses put forth in ethical codes, such as the *International Code of Nursing Ethics* and the ANA *Code for Nurses,* are binding on the nurse. The only time a nurse is excused from fulfilling any one of these duties is when doing so conflicts with fulfilling a more-stringent duty. As we have seen in the research example, how we determine which of several conflicting duties is the most stringent is a complicated issue that must be decided by an independent procedure (more on this later).

An obvious implication of following this procedural rule is that one must, in fact, be in a conflict-of-duty situation before one is relieved of any duties. If a strike could be conducted without violating any immediate responsibilities, such a course of action would be required. Certainly, in most situations ways can be found to minimize the failure to perform conflicting duties—for example, by directing non-emergency clients to other accessible facilities which provide nursing service and where nurses are not on strike, and by continuing to provide intensive care and emergency nursing sevices. A strike satisfying these conditions would not be morally objectionable. On the contrary, if a strike is the only means or clearly the most-effective way to change prevailing conditions that are incompatible with high-quality nursing care, then it is morally mandatory.

If other conditions obtain, it will be far more difficult to justify a strike. For example, if one were in a facility far from other facilities providing nursing care and a strike would leave many without the possibility of care, the duty to the public "here and now" might be the stronger duty. Or suppose a group of nurses has made a pledge to their employer not to strike or has signed a no-strike contract. Keeping that agreement is incompatible with strike action. Until 1968 the nursing profession (through the ANA) took a no-strike stance. The duty of fidelity (keeping agreements), which conflicts with striking in these situations, may also be one that cannot be outweighed by the duty to provide quality care to future clients. Fortunately, the ANA no longer adheres to a no-strike position, and most nurses are not working under no-strike contracts.

The moderate position defended here—condoning strikes in certain carefully circumscribed situations, claiming they are morally mandatory in others, yet not justified in still others—is a position that would be taken were nurses and the public to draw up an orginial contract. Consider the following hypothetical situation, following John Rawls, in which members of the public cannot know when or what nursing care they may need (they are under a veil of ignorance) (Rawls, 1971, 136–42) and nurses also do not know in what situation they will find themselves. Nurses as nurses would want to be able to provide the best care under the best conditions. They would seek sufficient power to be able to overcome any impediments to quality nursing care and self-respect. The public would be concerned to have available to them the best care possible within the limits of allocated resources. Under no conditions would they be willing to barter away a constant availability of emergency or lifesaving care. (They never know when such care may make the difference between life and death.) If it were determined that in some situations—due to factors outside the control of either nurses or the public—the only way quality care could be obtained would be by use of the strike weapon, nurses would insist on the right to use it, and the public would concur as long as emergency and lifesaving care could not be withdrawn. The public would agree to suffer the necessary inconveniences and hardship of a strike in the event that it were the only way to achieve high-quality nursing services.

The way to determine in a particular situation whether nurses' obligations to their clients and the public are weightier than the collective and future-oriented duty to take strike action is to appeal to the original contract. Would the public as party to the agreement be willing to make this required sacrifice in order to benefit from this sought-for goal? If so, the duties to one's clients or to the public that conflict with strike activity can justly be set aside in favor of the strike action. If not, they cannot.

Even if a strike can be morally justified, everyone would agree that it is an awkward and tortuous means of settling disputes. A better way would result from a three-party initial compact, a compact which also included the nurses' employers. Such an agreement would commit both nurses and employers to binding arbitration. That is, if a dispute between nurses and their employer could not be resolved by collective bargaining, it would be turned over to a mutually acceptable arbitrator. (The mechanics of this could be worked out in a variety of ways.) Strikes could be avoided while achieving the end of improved care.

Clearly, such an agreement would be advantageous to the public; they would not have to pay the price for the failure of other parties to reach an agreement. Nurses would also find this to be in their best interest. They could avoid being forced into the extremely awkward position of causing hardship or at least inconvenience to those whose interests they have sworn to advocate. Employers in the orginial position would also see that they stand to gain. They could not count on nurses' inability or disinclination to vigorously press their demands. Faced with the prospect of having to concede just as much or more to striking nurses than in binding arbitration, they would prefer binding arbitration. Everyone would avoid the loss of income and goodwill that inevitably results from a strike.

Of course, in the present real-life situation the employer's lot is quite different. He or she has little to gain by accepting binding arbitration. Perhaps through moral suasion employers will come to see that they ought to accept it. More likely, however, binding arbitration will be accepted only when it is in a particular employer's interests to do so. This will be the case if nurses are able to exact as many concessions from their employers by striking as would be possible through binding arbitration. Only strong, united action on the part of nurses will achieve such a break-through.

As client advocates, nurses should do all in their power to avoid strikes. But paradoxically, the best way to acomplish this is to be ready and able, in appropriate situations, to execute an effective strike.

8

Questions of Justice

Nurse Jackson was troubled. Mrs. Senex had applied for admission to the Happy Haven Nursing Home, a voluntary skilled nursing facility under religious auspices. Nurse Jackson had reviewed the medical record but there seemed to be no basis for admission. Mrs. Senex's score on the Multiple Factor Assessment Instrument was below the cutoff point for patients admitted. An initial diagnosis of a broken hip proved erroneous: the hip was merely bruised and was now recovering nicely. Still, Mrs. Senex did seem to be depressed and a bit confused. In the interview with her daughter, she offered no objection to the plans being made for her admission.

On balance, Nurse Jackson decided, there was no way to justify her admission ahead of other patients on the long waiting list for the home. When Nurse Jackson presented her conclusion to the administrator of the home, he nodded understandingly but replied, "Mrs. Senex has been a volunteer fund-raiser for Happy Haven and she's worked hard for this institution. Besides, her son-in-law, Judge Howard, told me this morning that she really can't handle things at home any more. The judge knows all about our home and he feels it's best that she be here." When Nurse Jackson left the administrator's office, she saw phone messages from people on the long waiting list. She felt more confused than ever [Moody, 1981, p. 6].

Admission to nursing homes is only one of many situations in which the issue of justice is raised in health care delivery. What is a fair way to distribute scarce resources? Should a vacancy in a nursing home or a bed in an intensive care unit be given on the basis of need, on the basis of past contributions, on the ability to pay, on a combination of these, or simply in order of application (first come, first served)? Setting aside the distinct possibility that in the case cited the administrator is simply trying to curry favor with the judge, he is appealing to the principle of merit (her past contributions) as the appropriate basis for distributing the scarce resource at their disposal, namely, a bed in the nursing home. Nurse Jackson bases her recommendation that Mrs. Senex not be admitted on a combination of need and length of time on the waiting list.

How to make these kinds of decisions fairly—one of the fundamental questions of justice—is the main subject of this chapter. We shall try to determine what criteria should be used in making these choices. It is beyond the scope of this book to develop a full-fledged theory of justice by which we can demonstrate that the criteria suggested are the correct ones. We shall, however, show that the suggestions we shall make are consistent with, and at least partially derived from, the ethical position outlined in Chapter 1.

Justice is the part of morality concerned with determining what is due to whom. The question of one's due can be raised in all areas of life. (a) In the economic arena we ask: What is a fair wage? (b) In the criminal system we ask: What should be done with violators of the law? What is a just punishment for this offense? (c) With regard to taxes and other burdens we ask: What should be required of various wage-earners? (d) With regard to benefits and common resources of the society (e.g., natural resources, parks, educational opportunities, research funds, police and fire protection, health care) we ask: How are the goods to be distributed? The very difficult underlying philosophical problem is to work out a unified theory and a basic criterion to determine one's due in all the areas. We shall limit our discussion to this last set of questions as they relate to health care.

In Chapter 1 we saw that equals ought to be treated equally. This is the formal principle of justice. If we fail to treat equals equally we fail to act justly. For example, if we give blue-eyed children the chance to get an education but deny it of all brown-eyed children we are not treating equals equally. We can readily agree to the unfairness here because we do not admit eye color as a relevant difference (that is, as a difference which warrants this different treatment). If we are going to treat children differently with regard to educational opportunity, we recognize that we must show that the different treatment is based on a *relevant* difference, e.g., need, ability to pay, ability to learn, past performance, residency, and so on.

These observations guide us to the heart of the debate, namely, to the question of what is a relevant difference, a difference that should make a difference. Pre-Civil War slaveholders recognized the formal principle of justice, and many felt the burden of showing that their very different treatment of slaves, as opposed to members of their own race, was based on a relevant difference. To show this they made claims that Negro slaves were genetically mentally inferior to whites. Of course, we know that these claims were and remain unsubstantiated. (And even if substantiated, it is not at all clear that it is a morally relevant difference.) The fact that they felt the need to make such claims, however, shows that even they realised that their difference of treatment required a defense to establish a basis for the difference of treatment.

If we are going to try to justify different treatment of clients—for example, admitting some but not others to the best nursing homes or giving expensive life-saving therapy to some but not to others—we too must show that the differences among clients are relevant ones. Let us hope that the differences we point to in order to justify our differences in treatment are better grounded that those upon which the slave-holders justified theirs. Clearly, if they are not, the differences in treatment that characterize our health care system are unacceptable.

In considering the justice of our practices in providing health care, several distinctions are helpful. One is a distinction between just procedures and just outcomes. Most of the time we cannot guarantee a just outcome even if we have adopted a just procedure. The exceptions are cases such as the following: Two children are to share a chocolate bar. We want each to have an equal portion. So we ask one child to divide the bar and tell her that the other child will be given first choice. The child dividing the candy will do her best to divide it in equal portions. In more complicated distributions perfect procedural justice usually is not feasible. Even if the procedure is just, the outcome may not be. Despite just procedures, for example, the outcome of a criminal trial or a disciplinary hearing for an employee may not be just.

A just outcome cannot be guaranteed for another reason as well, given the moral position defended in this book. We have emphasized the fundamental or preeminent role of autonomy in making moral judgments. As we have seen, autonomy often requires taking a hands-off position. Other autonomous agents may make decisions we cannot agree are fair. Yet if we are not to interfere (i.e., if we are to respect their autonomy), we must let the decision stand. Discussion of justice consistent with this view of the place of autonomy will primarily concern itself with just procedures. Just outcomes are to be seen as worthy ideals that frequently are beyond the moral agent's power to achieve.

In the case cited above, Nurse Jackson had a role to perform beyond that of bedside care. She was not deciding what was best for her client; instead she had to assist in determining whether Mrs. Senex was to become their client. The moral question of hospital or nursing home admission is one of fair allocation of resources. Whenever a resource would be helpful to more people than can have it, fairness requires that some procedure be devised to determine who shall get it and who shall not.

Often decisions made at this level are called microallocation decisions in contrast to macroallocation decisions, those made at the level of governmental bodies (e.g., decisions concerning how much to spend for medical research, or nursing education, or health maintenance organizations, or dialysis machines). Distinguishing, on the one hand, between these two levels (macro- and microallocation) of decision-making and, on the other, between allocation decisions at these levels and decisions at the bedside, is essential for clarity of thought. Considerations appropriate at one level are not appropriate at the others.

A health professional at the bedside should not be required to consider whether the use of a particular limited resource, which may help his or her client, is the best use of that resource. As Howard Hiatt has said:

A physician or other provider must do all that is permitted on behalf of his patient. In that sense, the physician is or should be responsible, with his patient and the patient's family, for setting priorities for that patient's management, within the limits available. The patient and the physician want no less, and society should settle for no less [Hiatt, 1975].

For a health professional to be able to care for her or his client in this fashion, allocation decisions setting priorities must already have been made on the administrative and governmental levels. If the physician or nurse is not going to be forced to decide case by case to whom to give the last pints of a rare blood type (e.g., to his or her elderly client or to a young accident victim), the administration of the hospital must have adopted guidelines and procedures for the distribution of limited resources. It is one thing for the administration (which may include health professionals) to make *general* policy decisions about the use of limited resources—for example, to decide that priority should be given to one type of client (a young person) over another (an elderly person) when both cannot be helped (due to a lack of resources). It is quite another thing for a health professional providing bedside care to make these judgments. These are decisions that must be made by category rather than in terms of individuals.

Of course, if the allocation decision by categories is to be fair, the difference in treatment of people in one category as opposed to another must be based on a relevant and defensible difference. Would age difference, to take the example cited, be a relevant and defensible difference? This, and other candidates for justifying different treatment, will be examined below.

Nurses and physicians may not want to go beyond the individualistic perspective of bedside care and may prefer not to consider the moral dilemmas of allocation of resources. This would then leave allocation decisions to others to determine the guidelines and limits within which the professional practices. Other health professionals may feel that these allocation decisions should be made exclusively by them. But since these decisions involve far more than questions of medical judgment, it is arbitrary to delegate them to one perspective at the expense of all the others. A more-reasonable attitude would be for health professionals to desire and to seek to play a role in the formulation of these policies. Whether we like it or not, health planning is done at the federal, state, and city levels of government. Elected and appointed officials quite appropriately calculate the benefits and the costs of alternative health policies and respond to political pressure from interest groups and lobbies. Although considerations such as these would be quite inappropriate at the bedside, they are a necessary part of democratic decision-making. The people through their representatives participate in the decisions concerning how their tax dollars are to be spent.

If the world had unlimited resources and all persons had unlimited sympathy for others, we could be spared these decisions (cf. Hume, 1888, pp. 490-500). But that people have limited sympathy for others and that we compete for scarce resources are beyond doubt. Specifically, dollars for health care must compete with dollars for defense, police and fire protection, education, roads, parks, and so on. Once a portion of our resources is set aside for health care, competition begins on another level between advocating funds for cancer research, hemodialysis, heart and lung diseases, improved nursing homes and facilities for the elderly and the chronically ill, preventive care, and better pay and working conditions for nurses.

Health care will always be a scarce resource. The more we can do (e.g., with plastic surgery, artificial limbs, organ transplantation, expensive diagnostic equipment) the more we want and the more we feel we are entitled to receive. Health care is a bottomless pit. The demand will always outstrip the available resources.

With these grim facts before us, we can understand why a popular analogy for our situation is that of the plight of a group of people adrift in an overcrowded lifeboat. Not all can be saved. The fundamental question becomes: is there any fair way to determine who shall be saved and who shall die? I think this is a reasonably good analogy to help us see what the fundamental test of a just procedure for making decisions in the allocation of health services would be. We must ask: Would the persons who lose out in the competition have grounds for complaint against those who made the decision? Of course, such persons will be disappointed. The question is whether, beside disappointment, they have grounds for complaint against us. Suppose we were to decide that all persons who belong to our own racial or national group will be saved but as many of the others as is necessary will be thrown overboard. Clearly, the latter group would have grounds for complaint. (The fact that they would have little opportunity to register their complaints compounds the injustice of our action).

The person in the overcrowded lifeboat who wished to act justly would seek a procedure which could be recognized as fair even by those who lost out in the competition. "Justice favours each man as much as is possible to do without being unfair to others . . . justice gives each man his due not merely reluctantly but of set purpose, and is reluctant only to have to disappoint the expectations of any man by arriving at a decision which is adverse to him" [Lucas, 1980, p. 18].

Being reluctant to act against anyone's interests but being required by scarcity to do so, the just person would seek a way that the disappointed persons could agree treated them with full respect and as equals. One method often suggested to satisfy the demands of justice is a lottery. In a lottery each person has the same chance as anyone else of being saved. It is argued that a procedure giving everyone an equal chance is consistent with the conviction that everyone is equal to every other individual in dignity and worth. The procedure also recognizes the rationality of each individual in that it is a procedure to which each rational person could agree. Hence, a strong argument can be made in favor of a lottery. Departures from a strict lottery would then require special defences: a case would have to be made that there were factors present that require us to treat certain groups of individuals differently from others.

Justice has two parts. It "demands not merely that we treat like cases alike, but equally important, that we treat different cases differently" [Lucas, 1980, p. 176]. We must determine not only whether equals are being treated equally but whether unequals are being treated differently. Only then is each person receiving his or her due. Someone might complain that in the lottery she was not given her due, that, for example, she should have been given special consideration because of her earlier contributions to the community. Is this an adequate reason to give her preferential treatment? Surely we cannot make an exception for her. (Then we would not be treating equals equally.) But suppose we adopt a policy that gives special consideration to *all* who have made substantial contributions to the community. (She may be the only member of the class of contributors. That just means that she is the only person possessing the relevant difference.) Would those who lose out in the competition have ground for complaint? This is a very involved question with the answer depending on such factors as whether the others had the opportunity to contribute but did not do so, and whether the individuals who did contribute did so merely because they, as a result of the luck of the draw (e.g., having received large inheritances), had more to give. These are precisely the issues raised by the case of Mrs. Senex's admission to the nursing home. Whether the others on the waiting list would have grounds for complaint if she were admitted ahead of them by virtue of her past contributions would depend on conditions such as these.

Suppose there were an agreement that service to the nursing home would be a factor in selecting people for admission, and suppose further that all potential candidates for admission to the home could volunteer to serve. These (unrealistic) conditions make it unlikely that candidates who are not selected have grounds for complaint on this score. Of course, it is unlikely in real-life situations (such as the case of Mrs. Senex) that these conditions obtain. This does show the procedure that must be followed, however, if we are to depart from selecting those in need of the service by a lottery. From what we have said it follows that justice does permit us to use criteria other than a strict lottery for discrimination among candidates for a benefit, as long as these criteria are ones to which we can rationally agree, they are known to be the criteria to be used, and no one is arbitrarily excluded from the competition for them.

It is important to stress that, were it not for the fact of scarcity, we could say—just as with lifeboats—that everyone in *need* of the resource must get it. Consider the following parallel siuation: There is an accident at sea; there are enough lifeboats for all aboard; but the crew just does not want to bother lowering more of them into the water. Each of them already is assured a seat. Clearly, only scarcity of lifeboats (or scarcity of time to get into them, and the like) would be sufficient ground for denying any passengers a seat. On the criterion of need alone, the same is true for health care.

If the *only* consideration that is morally relevant in determining who should get health care (or a seat in a lifeboat) and who should be denied it is need, then in a situation of scarcity (i.e., when there are more truly needy than can be helped) a procedure involving random selection is the only morally defensible way to decide who shall get health care. Nevertheless, I have been suggesting that, with certain conditions satisfied, there may be other factors as well which ought to be weighed. Let us consider a number of the most-plausible possibilities in addition to need. (Surely, as we have said, need is the obvious basis for distributing health care, leaving aside preventive medicine. The question is whether factors *in addition* to need may and ought to be considered.)

We have already considered the criterion of merit or past contributions. We saw that under specified conditions certain types of health care (e.g., early admission to a nursing home) could be allocated with past contributions factored in. The best analogy for this would be receiving a promotion for good work on the job. Yet this would hardly be appropriate as a criterion in providing health care to newborns, children, or the handicapped. If they lost out because they had not contributed, they have grounds for complaint. (Obviously they have had no opportunity.)

Perhaps, as some have suggested, in addition to need we should consider usefulness to society and potential for future contributions. Suppose, as was the case some years ago, we do not have enough dialysis machines for all who need them, and without access to the machines some will die. We have to decide how to distribute the limited resources. Each candidate has equal need. Suppose that those who are of most use to society win out because they score higher on this measure. The crucial question of justice is, do the losing candidates have grounds for complaint? Have they been judged by a standard that should not apply for the distribution of lifesaving therapy?

It seems that the answer must be that they have been judged by the wrong standard. This standard places higher value on the general good than on the integrity of the individual. The individual is being measured as a means to societal ends.

Only in very special situations (and most plausibly in those not involving matters of life and death) could one marshall a strong defense for the criterion of expected future contributions—as, for example, in North Africa in World War II when the scarce resource of penicillin was distributed to soldiers suffering from veneral disease rather than to those suffering from battle wounds. We can presume the Allies needed the able-bodied soldiers with veneral disease back on the battlefield as soon as possible. The wounded would not be able to return to battle for some time, if at all.

In an era of free-market capitalism, the ability to pay may seem a plausible criterion for determining who shall receive health care. If you afford the fee, you can obtain the service; if not, you cannot. Stated in this straightforward fashion, the criterion loses whatever initial appeal it may have had. Are we really willing to let someone with a ruptured appendix die because he or she is unable to pay? Suppose that everyone were endowed with the ability to earn sufficient income to pay for any basic health care need that arose. Yet some people foolishly spend their money on other things, gambling that they will not become ill. We can imagine someone arguing that these people made their choice, foolish as it was; now they must be willing to take the consequences.

Whatever one thinks of the argument, the assumption that everyone has the ability to earn sufficient income to pay for all basic health care needs does not square with the reality of our world. Circumstances—both individual misfortune (e.g., disability or exceptionally poor health, or a condition that requires costly treatment) and shortcomings of economic systems (e.g., the need for a certain percentage of unemployed workers)—place many in the group who are unable to pay for even basic care. Are we treating these people fairly if we withhold basic health care from them? Do they have grounds for complaint because they were denied care as a result of their inability to pay? Since, at least for people such as these, the inability to pay is not a result of circumstances within their control, to compound their misfortune by further deprivation seems not only lacking in compassion but surely is also grounds for their complaint.

In contrast, if the health care desired were not basic but sought to maintain an affluent life-style (e.g., hair transplants for bald men), the same basis for complaint cannot exist. We shall discuss the reasons for this later. For now we note that, although ability to pay is not an appropriate criterion for deciding who shall have basic, essential health care, it may be quite appropriate for nonessential care that aids one to maintain an affluent life-style.

We have looked at the ability to pay, usefulness to society, potential for future contributions, merit, past contributions, and need as criteria for determining who shall get basic health care or scarce lifesaving therapy. With the exception of need, the criteria examined were appropriate only in special, unusual, or extreme cases. In the vast majority of cases the one appropriate criterion is need. This seems to leave us, in cases of distribution of scarce resources, with some random procedure.

If we find that a random selection from the set of all those in need is less than satisfactory in certain areas of health care distribution and believe that the decision should be made on other bases as well, we must propose alternatives and see whether they could be accepted by disinterested, autonomous, and rational persons. For example, suppose that we were to consider adopting a policy that favors younger, healthier clients over elderly clients when the needed resource (e.g., the bed in intensive care, a life-support machine, blood, and so on) is scarce. Is this a policy we could agree to before we know what role anyone of us might play (that is, whether we will be young or old) in an actual situation? I believe that it is. Were we then to make widely known that this is the criterion for making distribution decisions in situations of scarcity, those who lose out and are disappointed would not have grounds for complaint. If we maintain that everyone has a right to a reasonably full life, we can support our decision to give priority to the younger person by arguing that the elderly person has already had one, whereas the younger has not.

Returning to the analogy of the lifeboat, suppose that having able-bodied sailors on each lifeboat would greatly enhance the chances of survival at sea. We could agree that the fact that a person is a sailor is a relevant factor. In addition, were it public knowledge that sailors needed to operate the lifeboats were to be given special status in a crisis, a person who did not get a seat would not have grounds for complaint on this score.

Effective and efficient emergency room care during a major catastrophe forces those providing care to discriminate among the victims by sorting them according to their medical needs (triage). There may be those who will die without immediate attention; for others it may be possible to delay treatment without immediate danger. Some may have only minor injuries; still others may be beyond help. Can we justify the different treatment which is the object of the sorting? The criterion for the sorting is need, clearly a relevant difference. Do those who lose out in the sorting (e.g., those not in immediate danger who have their treatment delayed) have grounds for complaint? I think not. But if each victim were treated simply on a first-come, first-served basis (one form of random selection), those who happened to be brought in later and had to wait but were in need of immediate attention would have grounds for complaint (were they still alive to register them). Although it would be an awesome responsibility no person would wish to bear, justice actually requires making these discriminations. The victims are different in terms of their need and, thus should be treated differently.

We cannot make the same distinction of needs in cases of shortages of life-support equipment when someone (any client including a defective newborn) with a poor prognosis is already on the machine and another client with a better prognosis and a better chance of benefiting from the machine is admitted. Here each client has the same desparate need for the life-support system. Since we would like to make the most-effective use of our resources, we may regret that the client with the poorer prognosis is already on the machine. But as long as the first client can benefit from the machine, we have no right to take it from him or her. We have made a commitment which cannot now be broken, even for the sake of another or for greater utility. To do so would allow the client to be used merely as a means to another's end. Of course, if the first client's conditions has worsened to the point that continuing on the life-support system is of no further benefit, then he or she should be removed and replaced by the second client. Tragically, the first client no longer needs the life-support system. His or her needs are for something greater that we cannot provide.

Continuing with the lifeboat analogy, let us return to another level of decision-making, namely, the decisions concerning how many lifeboats to have on board. If a ship's captain were to decide to set sail with only one-third of the lifeboats needed for all passengers, wouldn't this decision be one we would criticize? Suppose he agreed with the owner that it was just too costly to furnish all those lifeboats. Suppose they argue that to do so they would have to reduce the medical staff on board or make other equally undesirable cuts—otherwise they would make no profits at all. We are likely to be unconvinced by these claims because we feel that it is only fair that a space in a life-boat be provided for each passenger. This is protection to which each passenger is entitled. Still, we may more readily agree to other decisions that could lead to shortages of life-saving equipment or supplies. For example, we may feel we have no grounds for complaint if sophisticated medical equipment is not placed on board because it is thought to be too costly.

When there are items (as, for example, lifeboats) that we feel persons are entitled to—that is, that it is only fair or just that they receive them—we say that they have a right to them. In recent years especially, many have claimed that we have a right to health care. Clearly this statement is too vague. Yet there may be certain areas of health care we may consider to be on a par with that of the availability of lifeboat space for all passengers. If so, people would have a right to these.

Need is not only the primary basis for distribution of health care, it is also the basis upon which claims of a right to health care are made. The more fundamental the need, the stronger the claim that one has a right to it. The most-fundamental needs, needs that must be met in order to survive—food, water, air—are the least-controversial basis for asserting a right. Needs that must be met in order to live a life of rational activity, relatively free of pain, and so on, form a second level of needs. Examples are public education, immunization against debilitating diseases, eye glasses, hearing aids, and so on. From these needs for living at least a minimal quality of life we can move up to levels of needs required to maintain a luxurious life-style (e.g., hair transplants, certain cosmetic surgery). Defending a claim of a right needed to maintain the affluent life-style would be far more difficult (if not impossible) than defending the claim of a right to the items that satisfy the first- and second-level needs.

If someone has a right to something (e.g., to satisfy first- and second-level needs), this entails that others may not interfere with their obtaining it and that people in specified roles (for example, those in government) may have a duty to provide them. If we have a right to a certain level of care, a "decent minimum" (Fried, 1976), then—as we saw with the lifeboats—to deny it for cost reasons is unacceptable. Everyone must have full and equal access to that basic care.

Frequently, health providers are unhappy with the implications of these conclusions for the use and distribution of our national resources (e.g., the priority we must give to basic health care for the rural or inner city poor, as opposed to the many popular expenditures that really are indirect governmental subsidies of the wealthy) and that threaten the independence of health professionals (e.g., requiring nurses and doctors whose education has been subsidized by the government to practice for several years in an inner city or rural location). Unhappiness with the consequences of taking a moral position is not a sufficient reason to reject it. Promotion of one's own self-interest and preservation of one's favored status are not tests of moral adequacy. Concern for justice may require us to change our ways and even give up these things.

The objection to the claim that all persons have a right to a decent minimum of health care is often made in an exaggerated form. It is contended that the view is simply unrealistic; that our entire national budget would be given over to health care; and that many other areas of spending do far more than expenditures for health care to protect and promote life and health. For example, it is said, child nutrition programs, improved sanitation services, projects that clean our air and water, even certain crime prevention programs are likely to be more effective and efficient ways to protect and promote life and health than most health care expenditures. If we did have to sacrifice all these in order to support health care projects, it would, indeed, be foolish and an unacceptable outcome.

Were we in a situation in which resources were so limited that basic needs could not be met, then we, along with governmental officials, would have to make hard choices concerning which expenditures most effectively and efficiently protect and promote life and health. Happily, we are not at such a point. (Underdeveloped nations are faced with this problem. We who are fortunate enough to live in developed nations have a duty to assist them so that they no longer have to decide between death by starvation or disease for many of their citizens. But that is a subject for another book.) Nevertheless, even the wealthiest nations cannot afford every kind of technology and treatment that could be beneficial. For care beyond that which offers a context for a decent minimal quality of life for all, decisions based on criteria that include cost-benefit analyzes must be made. When choices must be made among the various possible beneficial programs (i.e., those that provide benefits above and beyond the decent minimum), these quite appropriately may reflect the will of the body politic.

Consider the following case:

State Bill 529 calls for the establishment of community-based homes for the care and education of the mentally retarded. The bill provides one home for every fifteen persons presently institutionalized in four state institutions for the mentally retarded at a cost of $55.8 million. The estimated costs for the new care for the present population of 7,600 will be $70 million a year.

The bill was introduced by Representative John Sheehan who spoke in favor of it. He painted a dismal picture of antiquated institutions bereft of basic human necessities or amenities. Thousands of human beings, many unclothed, spend their days huddled in dark, drab rooms, where they are supervised by an overworked staff, many of whom have no professional training. Sheehan, who has the support of the parents' organization, the State Department of Mental Health, the local ACLU, and the religious leadership, concluded his case by pleading, "Justice requires that we extend this token contribution to these citizens, burdened by physical and psychological suffering, and by the degradation of our society's past inhumanity to its fellow humans."

Representative James Hudson and Dr. Robert Simmons, while emphasizing their concern for the care of retarded, spoke in opposition to the bill. Representative Hudson, noting that he was elected representative of all the citizens in his district, argued that he had an obligation to examine the alternative uses for the $14 million in additional funds called for by the bill. But first, he pointed out that the new total sum of $70 million equalled 1.5 percent of the state's budget, a budget raised by all its citizens, while the institutionalized population equalled only one-tenth of one percent of the state's population. The proposed increase of $14 million could buy hot lunches for all the state's school children; it could also provide job training for productive members of society. Hudson argued that the fairest thing to do would be to spread the money evenly among those who would be productive. "Our task as legislators," he concluded, "must be to serve the greatest good of the greatest number."

Dr. Simmons, as a physician, argued that the money could be used more efficiently in providing health care for three groups: normal or more nearly normal children (thousands of whom could be reached for every mentally retarded child), those potentially engaged in productive labor, and pregnant women. He showed that much mental retardation can be eliminated through prenatal diagnosis which he estimated to cost $200 per case for Down's syndrome compared to $60,000 for each institutionalized child. Even allowing that some of the institutionalized retarded might be gainfully employed if they were in high quality, community-based homes, the savings from spending the funds on detection rather than on more expensive forms of institutionalized care are enormous.

The legislative committee must now make its decision on the bill [Veatch, 1975, p. 13].

Here we have three beneficial proposals but presumably sufficient funding for only one. Does justice require us to select one rather than the others? Clearly justice requires that something be done about the deplorable conditions in the antiquated institutions for the mentally retarded. These retarded individuals are being denied the basic minimum of care to which they are entitled. As we have seen, such needs must be met. The bill to establish community-based homes goes considerably beyond that basic minimum, however. It provides for desirable benefits, which undoubtedly would improve the quality of life of the mentally retarded. But the other suggestions for spending the health care budget also offer benefits that would enhance the lives of other needy groups (the undernourished, those under high risk of bearing defective children, the unskilled and unemployed). Individuals in these groups also are being denied the basic minimum that justice requires.

If we make certain that each of the needy groups is provided the decent minimum, and if (as may be the case here) we have additional resources to spend for health care, then we should select the programs that most effectively and efficiently improve the quality of life. Which program offers the most benefits relative to cost? These are the issues that must be resolved to make a decision in favor of one program over the others. Specific circumstances, how well each program has been devised, the support in the community for the different programs, and many other factors will have to be considered.

If a decent minimum is available to all (less than this cannot be morally defended) and additional funds are available for other health care projects, I have been suggesting we should carefully consider how we can most effectively and efficiently spend those funds to protect and promote life and health. In the past we have often failed to decide these issues by this criterion. Instead, special interest groups and organizations committed to exotic technological solutions frequently have won the budget battle. The most needy have been overlooked, while additional benefits have been showered on those already well supplied.

As special interest groups have gained support for exotic treatments to cure the diseases of affluence, the traditional functions of the public health nurse have been shortchanged. Education for self-help, prevention of the spread of disease, programs for education in nutrition, child care, and so on, have lost out to the interest of those in highly specialized and technical areas. The irony is that the conditions or diseases which the (impressive and valuable) exotic therapies are designed to ameliorate or, in some cases, cure are frequently the result of the lack of the preventive programs (including health education) once administered by public health nurses. Clearly, a more-efficient use of our resources would lead us to put more money into preventive care—public health nursing—and less into certain types of curative care.

Political realities (for example, the relative power of the American Medical Association, which emphasizes research and technology for advancing our ability to cure, in contrast to that of various nursing organizations, which would emphasize programs of prevention) make it difficult to move closer to a preventive care orientation. But even if these roadblocks were removed there would be other difficulties. One of these is that we can identify specific people who will benefit from projects that offer promise of cure of a particular disease; this is not the case for preventive care. We may know someone suffering from a heart condition, which could be corrected by open-heart surgery or a transplant. Our compassion pushes us in the direction of expenditures for particular suffering people. Preventive care is aimed at preventing the need for such help. Frequently there are no clearly identifiable persons who will benefit from the preventive care approach. For example, an effective antismoking campaign may prevent any number of people from smoking and developing lung cancer; but we do not know who will benefit or whose lives will be saved by the program. In contrast, if we effectively treat a smoker who has lung cancer; we help an identifiable person in need. As difficult as it is to do, efficiency often requires us to place greater emphasis on funding the more-impersonal preventive care programs than the exotic treatment to specific persons (perhaps afflicted with diseases associated with their affluent life-styles).

If nurses are going to take an active role on the institutional and governmental levels of decision-making, they would do well to emphasize their traditional concerns for preventive care and health care education and work as advocates of these programs. In this capacity nurses will be working as concerned citizens with special knowledge and training to back up their advocacy. Nurses are the key to both a more-just and a more-efficient national health care policy.

Bibliography and References

Abrams, N. 1974. "A Contrary View of the Nurse as Patient Advocate," *Journal of Nursing Administration* 4 (March–April): 40–44.

Ad Hoc Committee of the Harvard Medical School to Examine the Definition of Brain Death. 1968. "A Definition of Irreversible Coma." *Journal of the American Medical Association* 205, no. 6 (August 6): 337–40.

Alsop, S. 1971. "The Right to Die with Dignity." *Good Housekeeping*, August.

American Nurses' Association (ANA). 1976. *Code for Nurses with Interpretive Statements.* American Nurses' Association, Kansas City, Mo.

———. 1978. *Perspectives on the Code for Nurses.* American Nurses' Association, Kansas City, Mo.

Annas, G. J. 1975. *The Rights of Hospital Patients.* New York: Avon Books.

Aroskar, M. A. 1980. "The Fractured Image: The Public Stereotype of Nursing and the Nurse." In *Nursing: Images and Ideals,* edited by S. Gadow and S. Spicker, pages 18-34. New York: Springer Publishing Co.

Arras, J. D. 1981. "Health Care Vouchers for the Poor." *The Hastings Center Report* 11, no. 4 (August): 29–39.

Arras, J., and Jameton, A. 1979. "Medical Individualism and the Right to Health Care." In *Intervention and Reflection: Basic Issues in Medical Ethics,* edited by R. Munson. Belmont, CA: Wadsworth Publishing Co.

Ashley, J. 1977. *Hospitals, Paternalism, and the Role of the Nurse.* New York: Teachers College Press.

Baier, K. 1958. *The Moral Point of View.* Ithaca, N.Y.: Cornell University Press.

———. 1972. "Guilt and Responsibility." In *Individual and Collective Responsibility,* edited by P. A. French, pages 37-61. Cambridge, Mass.: Schenkman Publishing Co.

Baker, R. 1980. "Care of the Sick and Cure of Disease: Comment on 'The Fractured Image." In *Nursing: Images and Ideals,* edited by S. Gadow and S. Spicker, pages 41–48. New York: Springer Publishing Co.

Bandman, E. 1978. "How Much Dare You Tell Your Patient?" *RN* 41 (August).

Bandman, E., and Bandman, B. 1978. *Bioethics and Human Rights.* Boston: Little, Brown & Co.

Beauchamp, J. M. 1975. "Euthanasia and the Nurse Practitioner." *Nursing Forum* 14 (Summer): 56-73.

Beauchamp, T. L., and Childress, J.F. 1979. *Principles of Biomedical Ethics.* Oxford: Oxford University Press.

Beauchamp, T. L., and Walters, L. 1978. *Contemporary Issues in Bioethics.* Belmont, CA.: Dickenson Publishing Co.

Behnke, J. A., and Bok, S. 1975. *The Dilemmas of Euthanasia.* Garden City, N.Y.: Anchor Press, Doubleday.

Beletz, E. E. 1974. "Is Nursing's Public Image Up to Date?" *Nursing Outlook* 22, no. 7, (July): 432–35.

Benton, R. G. 1978. *Death and Dying: Principles and Practices in Patient Care.* New York: D. Van Nostrand Co.

Berg, D. L., and Isler, C. 1977. "The Right to Die Dilemma—Where Do You Fit In?" *RN* 40 (August):49–55.

Berwind, A. 1975. "The Nurse in the Coronary Care Unit." In *The Law and the Expanding Nursing Role,* edited by B. Bullough, pages 82–94. New York: Appleton-Century-Crofts.

Besch, L. 1979. "Informed Consent: A Patient's Right." *Nursing Outlook* 27 (January): 32–35.

Bleich, D., and Veatch, R. M. 1975. "Interns and Residents on Strike." *The Hastings Center Report* 5, no. 6 (December): 7–9.

Bok, S. 1978. *Lying: Moral Choice in Public and Private Life.* New York: Pantheon Books.

Brandt, R. 1975. "A Moral Principle About Killing." In *Beneficent Euthanasia,* edited by M. Kohl, pages 106–14. Buffalo, N.Y.: Prometheus Books.

Branson, H. 1972. "Nurses Talk About Abortion." *American Journal of Nursing* 72, no. 1 (January):106–9.

Brauer, P. H. 1960. "Should the Patient Be Told the Truth?" *Nursing Outlook* 8 (December): 672–76.

Brody, H. 1976. *Ethical Decisions in Medicine.* Boston: Little, Brown & Co.

Brooten, D.; Hayman, L.; and Naylor, M. 1978. *Leadership for Change: A Guide for the Frustrated Nurse.* Philadelphia: J. B. Lippincott Co.

Browning, M. H., and Lewis, E. P. 1972. *The Dying Patient: A Nursing Perspective.* New York: The American Journal of Nursing Company.

———. 1973. *The Expanded Role of the Nurse.* New York: The American Journal of Nursing Company.

Bullough, B. 1975. *The Law and the Expanding Nursing Role.* New York: Appleton-Century-Crofts.

Bullough, V. L. 1975. "Licensure and the Medical Monopoly." In *The Law and the Expanding Nursing Role,* edited by B. Bullough. New York: Appleton-Century-Crofts.

Callahan, D. 1970. *Abortion: Law, Choice & Morality.* New York: The Macmillan Company.

Campbell, A. V. 1975. *Moral Dilemmas in Medicine.* Edinburgh: Churchill Livingstone.

Carroll, M. A., and Humphrey, R.A. 1979. *Moral Problems in Nursing: Case Studies.* Washington, D.C.: University Press of America.

Cawley, M. A. 1977. "Euthanasia: Should It Be a Choice?" *American Journal of Nursing* 77 (May): 859–61.

Char, W. F., and McDermott, J. F., Jr. 1972. "Abortions and Acute Identity Crises in Nurses." *American Journal of Psychiatry* 128, no.8 (February): 952–57.

Chaska, N. L. 1978. *The Nursing Profession: View Through the Mist.* New York: McGraw-Hill Book Co.

Chudleigh, M. K. 1978. "The Nurse." In *Death and Dying: Principles and Practices in Patient Care,* edited by R. G. Benton, pages 241-53. New York: D. Van Nostrand Co.

Cleary, M. A. 1978. *1979 Medical & Health Annual: Encyclopaedia Britannica.* Encyclopaedia Britannica Inc.

Cohen, M.; Nagel, T.; and Scanlon, T. 1974. *The Rights and Wrongs of Abortion.* Princeton, N.J.: Princeton University Press.

Cooper, D. E. 1968. "Collective Responsibility." *Philosophy* 43, no. 165 (July):258–68.

———. 1972. "Responsibility and the 'System.' " In *Individual and Collective Responsibility,* edited by P.A. French, pages 81–100. Cambridge Mass.: Schenkman Publishing Co.

Creighton, H. 1977. "Action for Wrongful Life." *Supervisor Nurse* 8, no. 4 (April).

Daniels, T. 1979. "The Nurse's Tale." *New York Magazine,* April 30, 1979.

Davis, A.J. 1969. "Self-Concept, Occupational Role Expectation, and Occupational Choice in Nursing and Social Work." *Nursing Research* 18, no. 57 (January–February).

Davis, A., and Aroskar, M. 1978. *Ethical Dilemmas and Nursing Practice.* New York: Appleton-Century-Crofts.

Delora, J.R., and Moses, D.V. 1969. "Specialty Preferences and Characteristics of Nursing Students in Baccalaureate Programs." *Nursing Research* 18, no. 2 (March–April): 137–44.

Dock, L.L. 1912. *A History of Nursing,* vol. 3. New York: Putnam's Sons.

Dodge, J.S. 1972. "What Patients Should Be Told." *American Journal of Nursing* 72 (October): 1852–54.

Donagan, A. 1977. *The Theory of Morality.* Chicago: The University of Chicago Press.

Downie, R.S. 1972. "Responsibility and Social Roles." In *Individual and Collective Responsibility,* edited by P.A. French, pages 65–80. Cambridge, Mass.: Schenkman Publishing Co.

Durand, B. 1978. "A Nursing Practice Perspective." In *Perspectives on the Code for Nurses.* Kansas City, Mo.: American Nurses' Association.

Dworkin, G. 1972. "Paternalism." *Monist* 56, no. 1 (June): 64–84.

Ellin, J.S. 1981. "Lying and Deception: The Solution to a Dilemma in Medical Ethics." *Westminster Institute Review* 1, no. 2, (May): 3–6.

Engelhardt, H.T., Jr. 1975. "Ethical Issues in Aiding the Death of Young Children." In *Beneficent Euthanasia,* edited by M. Kohl, pages 180–92. Buffalo, N.Y.: Prometheus Books.

English, J. 1975. "Abortion and the Concept of a Person." *Canadian Journal of Philosophy* 5, no. 2 (October).

Evans, F.J. 1974. "The Power of a Sugar Pill." *Psychology Today,* April 1974.

Feinberg, J. 1968. "Collective Responsibility." *The Journal of Philosophy* 65, no., 21 (November 7): 674–88.

———. 1973. *The Problem of Abortion.* Belmont, CA.: Wadsworth Publishing Co.

Fields, C.M. 1980a. "What Kind of Education for Nurses?" *The Chronicle of Higher Education,* February 11.

———. 1980b. "Drive to Require Bachelor's Degrees for Nurses Seen Heading to Some Questionable Programs." *The Chronicle of Higher Education,* April 21.

Fost, N.; Chudwin, D.; and Wikler, D. 1980. "The Limited Moral Significance of 'Fetal Viability.'" *The Hastings Center Report* 10, no. 6 (December): 10–13.

Frankena, W. 1973. *Ethics.* 2nd ed. Engelwood Cliffs, N.J.: Prentice-Hall, Inc.

French, P.A. 1972. *Individual and Collective Responsibility.* Cambridge, Mass.: Schenkman Publishing Co.

Freund, P. A. 1977. "Mongoloids and 'Mercy Killing.'" In *Ethics in Medicine: Historical Perspectives and Contemporary Concerns,* edited by S. J. Reiser, A. J. Dych, and W. J. Curran, pages 536–39. Cambridge, Mass.: MIT Press.

Fried, C. 1976. "Equality and Rights in Medical Care." *The Hastings Center Report* 6, no. 1 (February): 29–34.

Gadow, S., and Spicker, S., eds. 1980. *Nursing: Images and Ideals.* New York: Springer Publishing Co.

Gaylin, W. 1973. "Patient Rights, Nursing Responsibilities." *Nursing Digest* 1 (October): 5–8.

Gillingham, J. B. 1950. "Collective Bargaining and Professional Ethics." *American Journal of Nursing* 50 (April): 214–16.

Godfrey, M.A. 1978. "Job Satisfaction—Or Should That Be Dissatisfaction? How Nurses Feel About Nursing." Part 1: *Nursing '78,* April 1978. Part 2: *Nursing '78,* May 1978.

Goldman, R. 1978. "The Social Impact of the Organic Dementios of the Aged." In *Senile Dementia: A Biomedical Approach,* edited by K. Nandy, pages 3–17. New York: Elsevier North-Holland, Inc.

Gorovitz, S., et. al. 1976. *Moral Problems in Medicine,* Englewood Cliffs, N.J.: Prentice-Hall, Inc.

Heidrich, G. 1980. "You Can Maximize the Placebo Effect of Every Treatment." *RN* 43, April.

Held, V. 1970. "Can a Random Collection of Individuals Be Morally Responsible?" *The Journal of Philosophy* 67, no. 14 (July 23): 471–81.

Hemelt, M., and Mackert, M. E. 1979. *Dynamics of Law in Nursing and Health Care*. Reston, Va.: Reston Publishing Co.

Hershey, N. 1970. "When Is a Communication Privileged?" *American Journal of Nursing* 70 (January): 112–13.

Hiatt, H. 1975. "Protecting the Medical Commons: Who is Responsible?" *The New England Journal of Medicine* 293, no. 5 (July 31): 235–41.

Hill, T. E., Jr. 1973. "Servility and Self-Respect." *The Monist* 57, no. 1 (January): 87–104.

Humber, J. M., and Almeder, R. F. 1976. *Biomedical Ethics and the Law*. New York: Plenum Press.

Hume, D. 1888. *A Treatise of Human Nature*. Edited by L. A. Selby-Bigge. Oxford: Oxford University Press.

Hume, D. 1957 reprint edition. *An Inquiry Concerning the Principles of Morals*. Edited by Charles W. Hendel. The Liberal Arts Press, Inc. Indianapolis, Ind.: The Bobbs-Merrill Co.

Ingelfinger, F. J. 1972. "Informed (but Uneducated) Consent." *New England Journal of Medicine* 287, no. 9 (August): 465–66.

Jameton, A. 1977. "The Nurse: When Roles and Rules Conflict." *The Hastings Center Report* 7, no. 4 (August): 22–23.

Jonsen, A. R.; Phibbs, R. H.; Tooley, W. H.; and Garland, M. J. 1975. "Critical Issues in Newborn Intensive Care: A Conference Report and Policy Proposal." *Pediatrics* 55, no. 6 (June): 756–68.

Kalisch, P.A., and Kalisch, B. J. 1978. *The Advance of American Nursing*. Boston: Little, Brown & Co.

Kaltreider, N.B.; Goldsmith, S.; and Margolis, A. J. 1979. "The Impact of Midtrimester Abortion Techniques on Patients and Staff." *American Journal of Obstetrics and Gynecology* 135, no. 2 (September): 235–38.

Kane, F. J.; Feldman, M.; Jain, S.; and Lipton, M. A. 1973. "Emotional Reactions in Abortion Service Personnel." *Archives of General Psychiatry* 28 (March): 409–11.

Kant, I. 1947 reprint. *Anthropology from a Pragmatic Point of View*. Translated by Mary J. Gregos. The Hague: Martinus Nijhoff.

Kant, I. 1949 reprint. *Fundamental Principles of the Metaphysic of Morals*. Translated by Thomas K. Abbott. The Liberal Arts Press, Inc. Indianapolis, Ind.: The Bobbs-Merrill Co.

Kastenbaum, B. K., and Spector, R. E. 1978. "What Should a Nurse Tell a Cancer Patient?" *American Journal of Nursing* 78 (April): 640–41.

Keller, C., and Copeland, P. 1972. "Counseling the Abortion Patient is More than Talk." *American Journal of Nursing* 72, no. 1 (January): 102–8.

Kelly, K., and McClelland, E. 1979. "Signed Consent: Protection or Constraint." *Nursing Outlook* 27 (January): 40–44.

Kelly, L. Y. 1978. "Nurse, Will You Tell?" *Nursing Outlook* 26 (February): 135.

Kohl, M., ed. 1975. *Beneficent Euthanasia*. Buffalo, N.Y.: Prometheus Books.

Ladd, J. 1979. *Ethical Issues Relating to Life and Death*. New York: Oxford University Press.

Langerak, E. A. 1979. "Abortion: Listening to the Middle." *The Hastings Center Report* 9, no. 5 (October): 24–28.

Levine, M. E. 1977. "Nursing Ethics and the Ethical Nurse." *American Journal of Nursing* 77 (May): 845–47.

Lewis, E. P. 1971. *Changing Patterns of Nursing Practice*. New York: The American Journal of Nursing Co.

———. 1977. "The Right to Inform." *Nursing Outlook* 25 (September): 561.

Lipman, M. 1971. "When Should a Nurse Blow the Whistle?" *RN* 34 (October): 54.

Lucas, J. R. 1980. *On Justice*. Oxford: Oxford University Press, Clarendon Press.

Maas, M., and Jacox, A. K. 1977. *Guidelines for Nurse Autonomy/Patient Welfare*. New York: Appleton-Century-Crofts.

McClure, M. L. 1978. "The Long Road to Accountability." *Nursing Outlook* 26 (January): 47–50.

McCormick, R. A. 1974. "To Save or Let Die: The Dilemma of Modern Medicine." *Journal of the American Medical Association* 229 (July 8): 172–76.

Mappes, E. J. K. 1981. "Ethical Dilemmas for Nurses: Physicians' Orders versus Patients' Rights." In *Biomedical Ethics*, edited by T. A. Mappes and J. S. Zembaty. New York: McGraw-Hill.

Mappes, T. A., and Zembaty, J. S., eds. 1981. *Biomedical Ethics*. New York: McGraw-Hill.

Mill, J. S. 1957 reprint. *Utilitarianism*. The Liberal Arts Press, Inc. Indianapolis, Ind.: The Bobbs-Merrill Co.

Moody, H. R. 1981. "Ethical Dilemmas in Long Term Care." *Human Values and Aging Newsletter* 3, no. 3 (May).

Munson, R. 1979. *Intervention and Reflection: Basic Issues in Medical Ethics*. Belmont, CA.: Wadsworth Publishing Co.

Nandy, K., ed. 1978. *Senile Dementia: A Biomedical Approach*. New York: Elsevier North-Holland Inc.

Navarro, V. 1975. "Women in Health Care." *New England Journal of Medicine* 292 (February 20): 398–402.

Noonan, J. T., Jr. 1970. *The Morality of Abortion*. Cambridge, Mass.: Harvard University Press.

Paige, R. L., and Looney, J. F. 1977. "Hospice Care for the Adult." *American Journal of Nursing* 77, no. 11 (November): 1812–15.

Pecorino, P. A. 1980. "Nursing Ethics, Technical Training and Values." *Process* 6, no. 2 (Summer).

Perkins, R. L. 1974. *Abortion: Pro and Con*. Cambridge, Mass.: Schenkman Publishing Co.

Plant, M. L. 1968. "An Analysis of 'Informed Consent.' " *Fordham Law Review* 36 (1968): 639–72.

Preston, R. P. 1979. *The Dilemmas of Care: Social and Nursing Adaptations to the Deformed, the Disabled and the Aged*. New York: Elsevier North Holland, Inc.

Quint, J. C. 1967. *The Nurse and the Dying Patient*. New York: The Macmillan Co.

Rachels, J. 1975. "Active and Passive Euthanasia." *The New England Journal of Medicine* 292, no. 2 (January 9): 78–80.

Ramsey, P. 1970. *The Patient as Person*. New Haven: Yale University Press.

Ratzan, R. M. 1980. " 'Being Old Makes You Different': The Ethics of Research with Elderly Subjects." *The Hastings Center Report* 10, no. 5 (October): 32–42.

Rawls, J. 1971. *A Theory of Justice*. Cambridge, Mass.: Harvard University Press, The Belknap Press.

Reich, W. T., ed. 1978. *Encyclopedia of Bioethics*. New York: The Free Press, a Division of Macmillan Publishing Co.

Reiser, S. J.; Dych, A. J.; and Curran, W. J. 1977. *Ethics in Medicine: Historical Perspectives and Contemporary Concerns*. Cambridge, Mass.: MIT Press.

Rescher, N. 1966. *Distributive Justice*. Indianapolis, Ind.: The Bobbs-Merrill Co.

Robertson, J. A. 1975. "Involuntary Euthanasia of Defective Newborns: A Legal Analysis." *Stanford Law Review* 27 (1975): 213–56.

Robinson, S. W. 1972. Opinion in *Canterbury v. Spence*, U.S. Court of Appeals, District of Columbia, May 19, 1972. In *Biomedical Ethics*, edited by T. A. Mappes and J. S. Zembaty. New York: McGraw-Hill.

Roe, A., and Sherwood, M. 1973. *Nursing in the Seventies*. New York: John Wiley & Sons.

Roemer, R. 1975. "Nursing Functions and the Law: Some Perspectives from Australia and Canada." In *The Law and the Expanding Nursing Role*, edited by B. Bullough. New York: Appleton-Century-Crofts.

Rothman, D., and Rothman, S. 1980. "The Conflict over Children's Rights." *The Hastings Center Report* 10, no. 3 (June): 7–10.

Russell, B. 1959. *Wisdom of the West*. London: Crescent Books.

Sandroff, R. 1980. "The Potent Placebo." *RN* 43 (April).

———. 1981. "Protect the MD . . . or the Patient? Nursing's Unequivocal Answer." *RN* 44 (February).

Saunders, C. 1973. "A Death in the Family: A Professional View." *British Medical Journal* 1, no. 5844 (January 6): 30–31.

Schlotfeldt, R. M. 1976. Editorial, "The Dependent Professional." *The American Nurse*, May 15, 1976.

————. 1978. "The Nursing Profession: Vision of the Future." In *The Nursing Profession: Views Through the Mist,* edited by N. L. Chaska, pages 397–404. New York: McGraw-Hill.

Selzer, R. 1975. "What I Saw at the Abortion." *Christianity Today,* January 16, 1976.

Shaw, A. 1973. "Dilemmas of 'Informed Consent' in Children." *The New England Journal of Medicine* 289 (October 25): 885–90.

Spicker, S. F.; Woodward, K. M.; and Van Tassel, D. D. 1978. *Aging and the Elderly.* Atlantic Highlands, N.J.: Humanities Press.

Stanley, L. 1979. "Dangerous Doctors: What To Do When the MD Is Wrong?" *RN* 42, no. 3 (March): 23–29.

Stein, L. 1967. "The Doctor–Nurse Game." *Archives of General Psychiatry* 6 (June): 669–703.

Steinbock, B. 1980. *Killing and Letting Die.* Engelwood Cliffs, N.J.: Prentice-Hall.

Steinfels, M. 1977. "Ethics, Education, and Nursing Practice." *The Hastings Center Report* 7, no. 4 (August): 20–1.

Sward, K. M. 1978. "An Historical Perspective." In *Perspectives on the Code for Nurses.* Kansas City, Mo.: American Nurses' Association.

————. 1980. "Precedents and Prospects for the Humanities in Nursing." In *Nursing: Images and Ideals,* edited by S. Gadow and S. Spicker, pages 3–17. New York: Springer Publishing Co.

Tate, B. L. 1977. *The Nurse's Dilemma.* Geneva, Switzerland: International Council of Nurses.

Tomich, J. H. 1978. "The Expanded Role of the Nurse: Current Status and Future Prospects." In *The Nursing Profession: Views Through the Mist,* edited by N. L. Chaska, pages 299–308. New York: McGraw-Hill.

Tooley, M. 1972. "Abortion and Infanticide." *Philosophy and Public Affairs* 2, no. 1, pages 37–65.

Veatch, R. M. 1975. "Case Studies in Bioethics: Case No. 529." *The Hastings Center Report* 5, no. 4 (August): 13–15.

————. 1976. *Death, Dying, and the Biological Revolution.* New Haven: Yale University Press.

————. 1977. *Case Studies in Medical Ethics.* Cambridge, Mass.: Harvard University Press.

————. 1980. "Professional Ethics: New Principles for Physicians?" *The Hastings Center Report* 10, no. 3 (June): 16–18.

Walters, L. 1974. "Ethical Aspects of Medical Confidentiality." In *Contemporary Issues in Bioethics,* edited by T. L. Beauchamp and L. Walters, pages 169–75. Belmont, CA.: Dickenson Publishing Co.

Warren, M. A. 1973. "On the Moral and Legal Status of Abortion." *The Monist* 57, no. 1 (January): 43–61.

Wasserstrom, R. 1976. "The Legal and Philosophical Foundations of the Right to Privacy." In *Biomedical Ethics,* edited by T. A. Mappes and J. S. Zembaty, pages 109–19. New York: McGraw-Hill.

Weir, R. F., ed. 1977. *Ethical Issues in Death and Dying.* New York: Columbia University Press.

Werner, R. 1974. "Abortion: The Ontological and Moral Status of the Unborn." *Social Theory and Practice* 3, no. 4, pages 201–22.

Wilson, H. 1974. "A Case for Humanities in Professional Nursing Education." *Nursing Forum* 13, no. 4.

Yeaworth, R. C. 1978. "Feminism and the Nursing Profession." In *The Nursing Profession: Views Through the Mist,* edited by N. L. Chaska, pages 71–77. New York: McGraw-Hill.

Young, E. W. D. 1978. "Health Care and Research in the Aged." In *Encyclopedia of Bioethics,* edited by W. T. Reich, vol. 1, page 65. New York: The Free Press, a Division of Macmillan Publishing Co.

Index

abortion: governmental funding for, 62; legalization of, 58, 67; nontherapeutic, 11; nurses' reactions to, 58–65; objectivity about, 63–64; on demand, 58; refusal to assist in, 59–62, 69–70; right to an, 61–62; and self-defense, 65, 69

accountability, 165

aged, the: and the need for care, 33–34, 99–111; and fair distribution of resources, 187–88

aging population, 33

aging process, 104

allocation decisions, 182–83; macro-, 182; micro-,192

Alsop, S., 86

American Medical Association, 136, 193

American Nursing Association, 163, 167, 171, 176

American Nursing Association *Code for Nurses*, 6–11, 14, 18–19, 31–32, 38, 39, 127, 164–65, 176

amniocentesis, 69

answers, 3, 5

appeal to authority, 14

applied ethics, 21

Aroskar, M. A., 31, 117, 122

Ashley, J., 30–31, 158

associate degree programs, 38

authority: appeal to, 14; assertion of, 53; clear line of, 43; final, 43; of health professionals, 121;

limits of, 54; of physicians, 46–47, 56; power and, 45–46

autonomy: attack on, 141; client, 36–37, 85, 88–91, 94, 97, 100–101, 103–4, 106, 111, 116, 119–21, 126–27, 134, 137, 144, 149, 150–51, 155–57; and deception, 139; disregard for, 142; and harming another, 152; justice and, 181; lack of, 144; limits of, 153; maximizing, 73; parental, 74, 76–77; principle of, 93–94, 104, 110, 112, 114, 131, 137–38, 146–47; respect for another's, 28, 54, 61, 148; restricting, 141; and utility, 153, 175; willingness to surrender, 128

autonomy, nurses': and abortion, 61–63; as special concern of, 44; and women's rights to have an abortion, 67

Baker, R., 31, 34

Barrett, M., 135

Beauchamp, T. L., 45

Beletz, E. E., 30

beneficence, principle of, 28–29, 175–76

Bentham, J., 25

Berwind, A., 33

binding arbitration, 178

Bleich, D., 174–76

Brandeis, L., 148

Brandt, R., 91